THE
FIT-OR-FAT® WOMAN

Covert Bailey
and
Lea Bishop

Houghton Mifflin Company / Boston

For information about permission to reproduce selections from
this book, write to Permissions, Houghton Mifflin Company,
215 Park Avenue South, New York, New York 10003.

Library of Congress Cataloging in Publication Data

Bailey, Covert.
The fit-or-fat woman / Covert Bailey and Lea Bishop.
p.   cm.
ISBN 0-395-50123-7
ISBN 0-395-51010-4 (pbk.)
1. Reducing exercises. 2. Exercise for women. 3. Women—Health
and hygiene. I. Bishop, Lea. II. Title.
RA781.6.B345   1989   89-30370
613.7′045 — dc19   CIP

Printed in the United States of America

BTA 10 9 8 7

Fit or Fat® is a registered trademark of Covert Bailey.

This one is for

CHRISTINA

so close, yet so far away

Contents

WOMEN ARE DIFFERENT!

Women and Their Fat

I DON'T KNOW which sex is fatter, men or women, and I'm not sure it really matters. I do know that fat is infinitely more damaging to women than to men. Women's hormones and habits urge their fat level up, while society urges their fat level down, and these opposing urges cause emotional conflict that most men can't even imagine.

In this book I will deal with the medical, the dietary, and the hormonal factors that drive fat up — and how to counteract them. But in the end, even the women who follow my advice will have more trouble with fat than men do.

Women seem to pay a much higher social price for their excess fat. Somehow, fat men "get away with it." Women are quite naturally upset that so much pressure is put on them to have perfect bodies. Much of their anger is directed at men, the Playboy centerfold, and male chauvinism. Their anger is understandable, but I believe the social pressures on women to lose fat come much more from other women than from men. A woman's appearance is not only scrutinized more carefully by other women but often unfairly criticized by the woman herself. "My breasts are too small, my thighs are too fat, my tummy should be flatter." One woman summed up the situation with the comment, "A compliment from a man is great, but compliments come easily from men. It really pleases me when a woman compliments me."

Women dress for other women. They may dress to please men as well, but usually it's what other women say that clinches the decision between the short skirt and the long skirt. Many women would be reluctant to go out in public if their husbands picked out their clothes.

Look at the mannequins used to display women's clothing. Are they realistic? Sweaters and blouses have to be pinned and gathered a ridiculous amount in order to fit them. A sweater small enough to "fit" a mannequin probably doesn't exist. Someone may claim that mannequins are manufactured to be skinny so that the shopkeeper can easily clothe them. Nonsense! Emaciated mannequins are like the super-skinny models in women's magazines. Somebody seems to think women ought to look that way.

Surveys of thousands of men and women have asked about preferences in women's (and men's) looks. The results clearly indicate that men do *not* prefer skinny women. Women seem to think that men like very slender legs, boyishly slim hips, and large breasts. The men surveyed, however, preferred larger hips, not boylike at all, but rather full. And yes, men like breasts, but much smaller than women imagine.

The surveys show that a man's idea of the perfect woman is much more realistic than a woman's idea. If we turn the discussion to men's bodies, we see the same kind of mistaken thinking. Men think that women want them to have huge shoulders and massive muscles, but most women prefer moderately muscled, athletic men. Movies featuring Arnold Schwarzenegger are watched by men, not by women.

The point is that much of women's frustration about body fat is a mistake. The desire for a super-skinny body is based on a misconception. But there is hope! A new idea is being born. The new woman wants muscles, a trim but strong body, breasts that don't impede her in athletics. Women who are fit are the new rage, and I have yet to meet a man who doesn't applaud them. As women exercise, their body fat decreases automatically, and their new muscles hold everything in place in the most pleasing way. Athletic women aren't often tricked by the skinny images in the media.

Watch out, everybody! The new woman is coming. She is free at last to have her own idea of how her body ought to look!

Women Get Fat More Easily Than Men

WHEN IT COMES TO FAT, women are behind that proverbial eight ball. Most fat men got that way by eating too much, but that isn't always true for fat women. I have counseled hundreds of fat women, and I am dismayed by their horror stories of starvation, sauna sweat sessions, appetite suppressants, and countless other gimmicks they've tried in order to do something — anything — to lose fat. Women get fat more easily than men, and it's harder for them to lose that fat. Let's look at the reasons why.

Male hormones keep muscle mass high and fat levels low. Female hormones tend to do just the opposite. Before puberty, the male/female differences are not so pronounced. Pre-puberty boys and girls that are normally active average 15 percent body fat. But when the hormones begin to flow, the girls' fat level climbs toward 22 percent. In contrast, the production of testosterone in boys results in a lowered fat level. By the time the two sexes are twenty years old, the fat level of active girls is 22 percent and that of active boys, 10 percent.

Many women supplement their natural hormones with artificial ones in the form of birth control pills. Put a man on birth control pills with no change in his eating or exercise habits, and in time he'll not only have more fat but he'll have it in the places where women tend to be fat. Female hormones alter metabolic pathways to favor the storage of body fat. The mechanism may simply be a reduction in the use of calories for heat and an increase in the use of calories to make fat. Women's metabolism tends to turn more of their calories into fat, while men's tends to produce more heat from calories. That's why your husband likes the temperature on his side of the bed lower than you like it on your side!

There was a time, about fifteen years ago, when your doctor would have scoffed at the idea that you could gain weight without increasing the calories in your diet. Medical schools used to insist, "A calorie is a calorie is a calorie. You can't gain weight unless you eat more of them." However, so many people gain weight when they quit smoking, it is obvious that you *can* gain weight with no increase in calories. Now we realize that weight gain occurs with hormones even if a woman *decreases* calories and *increases* exercise at the same time. The steroid pills that doctors often prescribe after menopause or hysterectomy, for example, seem to make women fatter even though their calorie consumption remains unchanged.

Women burn off fewer calories than men because their bodies are generally smaller and, more significantly, contain a lower percentage of muscle. A woman might weigh only 10 percent less than her husband but have 30 percent less muscle — and it's muscle that burns up most of our calories.

In their desperate attempt to get rid of fat, some women resort to fasting or to weird, unbalanced dieting gimmicks that simply worsen the problem. The effect of these gimmicks on body metabolism is devastating. Muscle is lost, and the body's ability to store fat increases. The body gears down and learns to function on a lowered calorie intake. These three factors working together make future fat gain almost inevitable and fat loss more difficult.

A woman's lifestyle adds the final frustrating straw. In today's society most women have two jobs, one outside the home and one at home. Surveys show that women still carry the greater responsibility in home chores. Additionally, women are not as sports-oriented as men; when they do have some free time, a game of tennis or a bike ride does not top their list of things to do. Lack of exercise also results in muscle loss.

In review, women get fat more easily than men because of four factors:

1. Female hormones
2. Less muscle
3. Unbalanced dieting
4. Lack of exercise

The first factor, hormones, is what makes you a woman. You'll always be a little fatter than a man no matter what you do. But you *can* do something about the other three factors, so read on!

First On, Last Off

MEN'S FAT DEPOSITS are so different from women's that the whole issue starts to get funny. Just think of the classic man with a big beer belly hanging over his belt. He probably has skinny legs under the fat belly, and his wife says, "I wish I had your legs." Men get fat the way a surgical glove blows up; their arms and legs stay skinny like the fingers of the glove while their bellies get round.

Women, however, tend to fill up like little tubs when they pour in the grease. That is, fat accumulates first in the thighs, then the hips and waist. Only when women are quite fat in their lower bodies does fat begin to accumulate under the arms and neck. And the process works the same in reverse. If you join a weight loss program, the first fat you lose will be from the neck and arms.

If a fat woman exercises on a stationary bicycle for six months, she probably won't have slimmer legs. She will actually lose more fat from her arms, even though it's a leg exercise. This is called the "first on, last off" rule. It doesn't matter what kind of exercise or diet she uses. Leg fat will not be reduced until upper-body fat is low.

A researcher once did years of work to prove that women with mostly upper-body fat are more likely to have diabetes than women whose fat is in their lower bodies. His conclusions seem ridiculous to me. If he had done body-fat testing on his subjects, he might have noticed that upper-body-fat women are simply fatter overall than lower-body-fat women. Upper-body-fat women are more likely to have diabetes because they have more fat.

Aren't we funny in our attitudes about our fat! Men scoff at women, women ridicule men, and we all just keep jiggling. Men hate their bellies, women hate their thighs, each sex thinks its fat is worse, and the battle goes on.

Is Your Mind Tuned In to Your Body?

OLYMPIC-LEVEL ATHLETES are incredibly in touch with their bodies, in tune with all parts of their bodies. A high jumper has to know exactly how high to lift her body to clear the bar without wasting effort on lifting any one part higher than necessary. Pole vaulters must do a similar thing. It is hard enough to lift the entire body sixteen feet in the air without adding an extra inch for one extra piece of anatomy.

Highly trained female runners on treadmills, hooked up to monitors of their heart rate, pulse, blood pressure, temperature, and brain activity, can often tell the researchers conducting the experiment exactly what the monitors are showing without seeing them! They are able to quite accurately predict how much faster they can go before collapsing in exhaustion. Women without such training, under similar circumstances, have little sense of where they are in relation to their abilities. The average woman running close to her maximum may feel that she can do no more; if pushed, however, she may actually run quite a bit more. Or she may tell the researchers that she feels great — but then she falls off the treadmill in the next few moments. Marathon runners develop the ability to pace themselves. If they have to abort the race in midcourse they are rarely surprised. Ordinary runners *are* surprised by such setbacks as well as by their successes.

The point is that a trained athlete has learned to connect her mind to her body's performance. She is in tune with her body on both a conscious and an unconscious level. As a person's physical ability or fitness level diminishes, this mind-body connection decreases. In very fat, out-of-shape people, the disconnection becomes obvious.

This disconnection is particularly strong in women, especially in fat women. Traditionally, women spend a lot of time ministering to the outward appearance of their bodies and less time on the muscles inside. Ten-year-olds, both boys and girls, put tremendous amounts of time and effort, through play, into developing their bodies. They keep fat down without even thinking about it. As adults, however, women are likely to dismiss their physical abilities and concentrate more on their appearance. They learn at an early age how readily looks can be altered. Unfortunately, fat on the outside is a manifestation of something wrong with muscle metabolism on the inside.

Some readers will think that I don't understand the tremendous pressures put on women to be beautiful. Believe me, I *do* realize it. It's sickening that both men AND women label others by numbers, saying "She will never be a 10." I, too, would feel terrible if the men and women I met reacted primarily to my looks instead of to the real me.

Sadly, women's magazines perpetuate the problem by showing unrealistic, skinny models. They do as much damage in upholding the "body beautiful" myth as do the voluptuous *Playboy* centerfolds. In other words, it's not all male chauvinism; women themselves augment the problem.

Let's accept that female beauty is important. Women *are* going to be judged by their looks. But what about lasting looks? What about the qualities that make relationships last? Consider all the beautiful women who are unsuccessful in relationships. Of all the male-female breakups, how many were caused by the woman's lack of beauty? Ask marriage counselors what causes divorce — it's rarely a lack of good looks. Marriages last or fail because of people's inner qualities. Are you letting your concern for looks take over?

Whether a woman reacts to attention by decorating her body or by abusing it, she becomes less and less in tune with what is going on inside. She views fat as something that has been tacked on. Diets seem to remove fat, so women use them as nonchalantly as they use nail polish remover. The muscles and their job are forgotten, and she becomes less active. Metabolism gradually decreases as fat increases.

Women need to concentrate on exercise and muscle to get in tune with what their bodies can do. Women's preoccupation with appearance disconnects them from the largest single facilitator in losing unsightly fat — MUSCLE. Get reconnected to your inner body. Make your muscles useful again. Push aside the idea that beauty is everything. Exercise will help you be everything that you can be, lowering body fat the proper way, making your skin and eyes and personality glow from the inside.

Healthy Women Do Jiggle!
Correct Body Fat Levels

ADULT WOMEN with less than 22 percent body fat represent a small fraction of the female population. It seems that 22 percent fat is a natural and healthy percentage for women with normal hormone levels and moderate *playtime* exercise programs. Staying below 22 percent fat seems to require rigorous exercise and diet for most women. Although it isn't completely accurate, I am inclined to think that only women who are professionally involved in exercise have lower fat levels. We have tested hundreds of Jazzercise instructors and have found that their average fat level is 18 percent. Women marathon runners who compete regularly average 18 percent — less if they are young, more if they are over thirty. Women over thirty who run and train enough to be able to complete one marathon often have more than 22 percent fat.

An interesting study was made of a team of women mountain climbers. Each woman in the group had previously climbed in the Himalayas to altitudes over 18,000 feet. Each of them was actively training for an assault on Annapurna. Most people would expect these women to be quite low in fat. Yet in this very tough group, the average body fat was 21 percent.

What do all these numbers imply? The average woman is extremely unlikely to be below 21 or 22 percent fat! And at this fat level, SHE WILL HAVE SPOTS THAT JIGGLE! If a woman's body fat is around 18–22 percent, some areas of her body, particularly the hips and thighs, will have extra fat. The buttock and thigh muscles may be quite firm, but most women, unless they are very young or have inherited thin legs and hips, carry a wiggling layer of fat in that area. Even super-athletic women — those who play professional tennis or run marathons — are not as solid in the hips and thighs as their moderately active male friends. This is simply part of being a woman.

If these women exercise a lot, watch their diet, and measure 18 percent body fat, how come they still jiggle? Let's do a little arithmetic. If a one-hundred-pound woman has 15 percent body fat, that comes to fifteen pounds of fat. Picture a pound of fat as a one-pound carton of butter resting on your kitchen counter. Now add fourteen more pounds of butter and think how big a pile of fat that is. Next try to imagine pushing those pounds of fat onto your body. Where would you put them? Most women could put one pound into each breast — perhaps two for large-breasted women. There are probably two pounds of fat around the intestines, another three pounds under the skin. Finally, put four pounds on the back of each thigh, and you've just about got it. Most women are way over 15 percent and have way more than fifteen pounds of fat. So Ms. Average Woman has another ten to twenty pounds under her skin.

The average woman I test is 30 percent fat, and she is more conscious of diet and exercise than most American women. To get from 30 percent to 22 percent is a large task; it is unrealistic to assume that you can easily reach the 18 percent dance instructor level. We advise people to work for ½ percent fat loss per month. To drop from 30 percent to 22 percent requires about sixteen months — and that's if you stick to a low-fat, low-sugar diet plus daily aerobics the whole time without falling off for two months in the middle.

Too many women, having learned that diet is not enough and that exercise is the only way to have a trim body, expect to get to 22 percent in less than one year. That doesn't seem realistic, considering the data above, showing that professional women athletes have between 18 and 20 percent. Olympic women figure skaters average 16 percent, and Olympic level gymnasts, 14 percent. Keep in mind that these women are on average seventeen years old. If you have gotten to 30 percent fat and are thirty years old, you have a lot of work ahead of you.

If all this has depressed you, take heart, because many other delightful body changes may come before you start losing weight. Start an exercise program today, and within a week you will feel the results. You will sleep better, getting more sleep *rest* from

Women's Body Fat Percentages

68%	Fattest I've tested
33%	Average American woman (my guess)
30%	Average at my clinic
27%	Healthy woman on estrogen after menopause or hysterectomy
25%	Healthy Oriental
23%	Healthy woman on birth control pills
22%	Healthy Caucasian
19%	Healthy black
18%	Aerobics instructor
	Long-distance runner
	Young girl (before puberty)
	Ballet dancer
	Professional athlete
	Body builder
10%	Gymnast
6%	Leanest I've tested

fewer sleep hours. A biopsy of your thigh muscles would demonstrate an increase in fat-metabolizing enzymes. In a month you will maintain your body temperature better, so that you need fewer layers of clothing on cold days. In three months emotional stress will seem to decrease as hunger control increases. In four months you can double your body's ability to metabolize fat.

Yes, it *is* hard to get body fat down, but you can reap many of the benefits of exercise right away. Personally, all I care is that my body fat is lower next year than it is this year. If you're fat, it probably took you several years to get that way. Reversing the trend is hard work and will take some time.

Dangerously Low-Fat Women

I'VE TESTED THOUSANDS of women in my water tank. Some of them were so fat and floated so well I couldn't do the test. But of the ones I *was* able to submerge, the fattest weighed 260 pounds and had 68 percent fat. Over two-thirds of her body was fat. Her comment was, "Wow! I wonder how fat I was last year *before* I lost 100 pounds!" I will come back to this woman — let's call her Madame X — in a minute.

The lowest-fat woman I've tested was 6 percent. Ann-Marie was an athlete but wasn't obsessed with sports. She loved tennis, playing several hours a day just for fun. She was also a great racquetball player, did a lot of bicycling, but only ran when there was "nothing else to do." She weighed 125 pounds and had a lovely figure, not too thin or too muscular. All her hormone levels were normal and her menses were normal. Ann-Marie isn't famous, but she ought to be.

In between Ann-Marie and Madame X are the more "normal" women that I test, who average 30 percent fat. These are women you see every day grocery shopping, running errands, going to work. They look a little overweight but not remarkably so. At 30 percent, they've added ten to fifteen extra pounds of fat, and although they may be unhappy with the way it looks, they seem to be just fine. As they shed those pounds of fat, these women do better and better. They play with their families more, they sleep better, they work harder, and, most important, they feel good about themselves. Because they feel and look better and better as their fat drops, however, some of them jump to the conclusion that the lower the fat, the better. Not so! Women who are between 18 and 25 percent fat seem to be healthiest physically and emotionally.

Too many women fall into the trap more typically associated with men — if one beer is good, two would be better; if less fat is good, no fat at all would be wonderful. As with most great ideas, we take a good thing too far. The joke in my office is, "The brain is made of fat, so if you get down to zero percent, you should become a politician."

Kidding aside, how low in fat is too low? We know that Madame X, at 68 percent fat, is courting medical disaster. What about 6 percent Ann-Marie at the other end of the scale? Is she super-super-healthy because low fat is supposed to be good, or is her fat level too low for good health? Many researchers claim that 6 percent fat in women is dangerous, partly because low fat causes menstruation to cease. Not so!

A study was done of female distance runners of similar age, height, weight, fitness level, and training schedule. The women were divided into two groups: those with regular menstrual periods and those who were quite irregular or weren't menstruating. The researchers wanted to prove that the nonmenstruating group was much lower in body fat. To their surprise, both groups had nearly identical body fat levels, averaging 17 percent. In fact, one of the amenorrheic women was 28 percent fat! They concluded that, although nonmenstruating women may have low body fat, it is not necessarily the *cause* of amenorrhea.

This and other experiments show that women may experience amenorrhea when there is a *sudden* change in body fat or body weight. Any powerful stress, whether emotional or physical, can trigger this reaction. Women in active war zones often stop menstruating.

Low body fat does not *cause* amenorrhea. Stress and sudden change do. It is true that amenorrhea in young women is associated with low estrogen production and with an increased likelihood of uterine cancer, breast cancer, and bone loss. Amenorrhea during the child-bearing years is very serious and is *associated with* low body fat. The question is, does low body fat *cause* the halt in estrogen production and the resultant amenorrhea? Probably not. Ann-Marie, at 6 percent, has normal female functions. She maintains low body fat without shutting off her ovaries. In other words, some women, like Ann-Marie, inherit a tendency to low body fat that IS NOT STRESSFUL for them.

It's not the level of body fat that is so critical, it's the effort required to get there and stay there. Let's suppose that 6 percent Ann-Marie has a natural set point of 12 percent. Her body, without any training, may fluctuate around the 12 percent level. She might be able to eat quite carelessly without gaining fat. Active girls aged twelve to fourteen average 15 percent fat even though they eat anything and everything. For these naturally low-fat females, a drop to 7 or 8 percent isn't so dramatic. For them to stay there isn't so dramatic either. For the average adult woman, however, it's a stress to get to such low fat levels and a stress to stay there.

When this subject comes up at my seminars, I am sometimes confronted by a woman who angrily points out that she is absolutely healthy in spite of having 8 percent body fat. She interprets the facts about low body fat as a direct insult. She's missed my point completely. It's possible to be very low in fat and be very healthy, like Ann-Marie. But such women are the exception. What I want to emphasize is that if your body stubbornly remains at 18–25 percent fat in spite of exercising three to six hours a week, eating a low-fat, high-fiber diet, then maybe it is trying to tell you something. Maybe it's saying, "Hey, I'm doing just fine. Don't mess with me!" If you attempt to push your body down to an abnormally low fat level it may retaliate by saying, "She's trying to get down to a man's fat level. I wonder if she wants to be more like a man?" So it stops menstruating, gets rid of all that fatty breast tissue, and perhaps even grows a small moustache!

The key, then, to good health in extremely low fat individuals is that they have taken a long, long time to get there and have inherited a low-fat tendency, like Ann-Marie. The scare stories about the danger of being too low in body fat are inappropriate. Low fat in itself isn't dangerous! The ovaries manufacture estrogen/progesterone from dietary fat. If you live on a severely limited diet, with strenuous exercise, crammed into a stressful lifestyle, you are adding three stresses together. Chances are the ovaries will not do their job on a regular basis.

I hope this information is startling enough to scare women a little, to prevent them from pursuing extreme low fat obsessively. I also hope that people will stop saying that very low fat in women is dangerous. Lots of stress is dangerous, not low body fat.

BEGONE, FAT!

How Do I Get Rid Of My Fat?

SUPPOSE YOU WOKE UP one morning to find that your hair was turning purple. Would you think, "Oh dear, my hair is turning purple. I'd better get something to change the color to its normal shade"? Of course not! You'd be alarmed and would want to know what's going on inside that's turning your hair purple. Yet when you notice you're getting fat, the usual reaction is, "Oh dear, I'm getting fat. I'd better go on a diet to get rid of it." Most people don't ask what is causing them to get fat. They only want to get back to "normal."

I'm not saying it's bad to go on a diet if you get too fat. What I am saying is that EXCESS FAT IS NOT THE PROBLEM. It's a *symptom* of the problem. The problem is, WHAT MAKES YOU GAIN FAT EASILY? You can call it metabolism, biochemistry, systemic health, or just plain fat chemistry. Use any phrase you like, but be sure to concentrate on the internal reasons for your fat, not on the external fat itself.

Having a cold is more than just a runny nose; it's fever, headache, coughing, congestion — a problem for the whole body. An antihistamine may lessen the symptom of a runny nose, but it doesn't cure the cold. Similarly, excess fat is a visible manifestation of an underlying systemic disorder. You can decrease fat, a symptom, with dieting or with surgery, but you haven't changed your metabolism or your tendency to get fat.

To focus on losing fat without doing something about changing your body's systemic tendency to get fat is akin to the purple-haired woman applying hair dye without doing something about why it's turning purple in the first place. So a sensible weight loss program must include a heavy commitment to making alterations in fat chemistry.

Some weight loss gimmicks, such as wiring the jaws shut, stapling the stomach, and taking laxatives, are so short-sighted and destructive that I won't waste time dealing with them. But other techniques, primarily unbalanced and/or very low calorie diets, are very widely used because people lose weight so quickly on them. I do not recommend these diets because they ignore the issue of metabolism. The classic example is the high-protein, low-carbohydrate, low-calorie approach (Atkins Diet, Stillman Diet, Drinking Man's Diet). Dozens of diets are based on this formula because weight loss is so rapid. Much of the weight lost is water, which is quickly regained, making the initial loss much less dramatic. Fat loss *is* quick with these diets, *but* there is also a significant decrease in the amount of body protein as reflected in muscle loss and in the loss of fat-burning (protein-structured) enzymes throughout the body. It's a superficial dietary manipulation that overlooks the long-term effects of muscle loss. After this kind of diet, fat control becomes more difficult, and over time people gain fat faster than ever.

I recommend a three-pronged approach to fat control:

1. *Aerobic exercise* to enhance the body's ability to burn fat
2. *Balanced dieting* to get rid of the symptom: excess fat
3. *Weight lifting/body building* to increase fat-burning muscle and shape body contours

Aerobic exercise burns very little fat during the exercise itself, and it stimulates only a slight increase in muscle, but it has *tremendous* effects on the metabolism of fat, on heat production (which uses calories), on fat cells, and on practically every other facet of fat chemistry in the body.

Aerobic exercise is by far the most important part of weight control because of its long-term effects on nearly every aspect of body fat, including the hunger mechanism, storage in fat cells, the ability of muscle to burn fat, and the brown fat mechanism. It has a *positive* effect on metabolism. Anyone who omits aerobic exercise from a fat control program will fail in the long run. You may control your weight by diet alone for a while but eventually you will have to eat less and less as your fat-burning metabolism decreases.

Balanced dieting is the second part of a good weight control or fat control program. It induces only gradual fat loss but it helps keep muscle from decreasing as fat decreases.

Weight lifting or body building is the last part of our program. In the past we did not include it because almost no fat is burned during the actual weight lifting. However, the changes in muscle do have a long-term effect on body chemistry by:

- increasing the amount of muscle so that the body uses more calories;
- improving posture and attitude. Physical strength seems to improve emotional strength;
- "waking up" deep muscle levels so that more muscle gets involved during aerobic exercise; and
- changing body shape. Aerobic exercise and dieting reduce body fat, but body building enhances curves.

Aerobic exercise and balanced dieting are dealt with intensively in my previous books *Fit or Fat?* and *The Fit-or-Fat Target Diet*. I recommend that you study them for background education. The following chapters of this section answer many of the questions about exercise and diet that weren't addressed in the first books. In addition, the chapter "How to Gain Weight" gives my rationale for weight lifting.

Exercise Advice for the Beginner

THE STRONGEST ADVICE I can give the beginner is to exercise often. Lots of articles in magazines state that maximum benefits are obtained by exercising three times a week, an hour each session. Such statements are misleading. Moderately fit people can do fairly well with such a schedule, but not the beginner. Aerobic exercise instructors love this advice because it fits their class schedules. But the advice doesn't fit high-level athletes who need much, much more than three hours a week, and it doesn't fit the beginner. Beginners should not exercise for an hour without stopping. And they should not limit their sessions to three times a week. Instead, they should exercise three or more times *a day,* for fifteen to twenty minutes at a time.

The neophyte's body isn't used to exercise. Doing three or four fifteen-minute sessions a day instead of one long bout not only makes you feel less tired but also seems to stimulate the body to initiate the various changes I described in earlier chapters. As you become more fit, longer sessions produce better results, but in the beginning I urge you to stick with short, frequent sessions. At times I do this myself, even though I have exercised all my life. On cold winter days when I'm at home writing in my study, I turn the heat down and hop on my stationary bicycle every hour or so. Pedaling for ten or fifteen minutes warms me up for the next hour and makes me feel more alert. I profit in three ways: I get fit; being alert helps me write more efficiently; and I save on the gas bill!

Beginners benefit from exercising seven days a week. The experienced athlete does just as well with fewer sessions, but not the beginner. Like a new puppy that hasn't been housebroken, the untrained body has to be constantly reminded with exercise before it starts behaving the way it should.

People often ask whether it's better to exercise in the morning or in the evening. Some studies have shown that morning exercisers are less likely to quit than those who do it in the evening. Other people claim that it doesn't matter when you exercise as long as you do it at the same time every day. They say that your body seems to prepare itself for the exercise by elevating temperature and heart rate, as if all the muscles were "warming up." I think morning versus evening versus same-time-of-day arguments are silly. The real issue is to make exercise fit your lifestyle. My lifestyle allows me to exercise at various times during the day, which I prefer because I don't get bored.

As a beginner, you should select at least one indoor and one

Do you have a friend who won't exercise because she believes in the wacky idea that each person has only a certain number of heartbeats in her lifetime and that exercise will use up these heartbeats prematurely? Tell her that exercise *lowers* the resting heart rate an average of 10 beats per minute. That's a saving of 600 beats an hour, over 14,000 beats a day! If you exercise thirty minutes a day at a heart rate of 140 beats a minute, you're only using up 4200 beats, leaving you a net saving of almost 10,000 beats a day.

outdoor exercise. There are many to choose from, and in *Fit or Fat?* I discussed the merits and disadvantages of several. Rather than reviewing them again, here's a quick selection. New readers can refer to the earlier book for more details.

Outdoor Exercises for the Beginner	Indoor Exercises for the Beginner
Walking/walking with hand-held weights	Stationary bicycle
Slow jogging	Rowing machine
Bicycling	Treadmill
Mountain hiking	Stair climbing
Cross-country skiing	Cross-country ski machine
	Video aerobic classes
	Aerobic dance classes

I especially recommend aerobic dance classes for women. They're fun, and they offer a camaraderie that encourages the beginner to stick with it. Because of the variety of movements and exercises, the beginner is less likely to experience the problems (shin splints, sore ankles, hips, and knees) associated with other, more repetitious kinds of exercise.

As a beginner, you have options that a fit person who exercises for longer periods might not consider. You can park a half mile from work and walk the extra distance in ten or fifteen minutes. While dinner is in the oven, you can sneak in twelve minutes to walk or slowly jog around the block. One woman I know wears a small backpack, walks one mile to the store, and, European style, buys just the groceries she needs for the day. In a way you have an advantage over the experienced athlete who has to make time to exercise. It's easy to slip in ten minutes here and fifteen minutes there.

You may also wish to do something *an*aerobic for your muscles, such as sit-ups, or you may want to exercise by playing a game such as golf; but be sure to do *aerobic* exercise for fat control.

After all the exercise discussion in this book, we need a clear definition of aerobics so that you won't buy a gismo or program that doesn't yield aerobic benefits.

An Exercise Program Is Aerobic If It

1. Uses the large muscles in the lower part of the body (buttocks, thighs), because working the big muscles has *systemic* effects.
2. Gets you warm and breathing heavily without being really out of breath and without producing lactic acid. This means your heart rate is 65–80 percent of its maximum.
3. Goes on without interruption for twelve minutes if all the muscles are used, as in a rowing machine or cross-country skiing; or thirty-five minutes if very few muscles are used, as in walking. The more muscle used, the less time it takes to get a systemic response.

Susan

WHEN SUSAN FIRST VISITED my clinic, I had the urge to bow down and kiss her hand. Her stunning face, warm complexion, and tall, regal bearing indeed gave her a majestic quality. From the neck up, Susan was gorgeous! Her auburn hair was accented by the golds and browns of her well-tailored suit.

So skilled was she at drawing attention to her good features that I was amazed when she blurted, "Covert, you've got to help me! I need surgery, but I weigh 200 pounds and I smoke, and my doctor won't operate until the cigarettes and pounds go." Susan had had knee problems for a number of years, and surgery was now necessary, but her physician rightly wanted her to do everything possible to ensure a quick recovery. Excess fat makes operating much more difficult, and smoking retards tissue repair. Many physicians refuse to do *elective* surgery until these two factors are under control.

When I spoke with Susan's physician, he agreed to a six-month delay of the surgery. During that time he recommended a low-intensity exercise program to strengthen the muscles around her knee. Any exercise was fine as long as she didn't overstress the knee area.

Susan, five foot nine and 196 pounds, was 36 percent fat. She had an eye for fashion, and her size 20 wardrobe well hid her 46-

inch hips and 28-inch thighs. She had been trying to lose weight — with little success — by skipping breakfast and having only soup for lunch. She would have one drink in the evening followed by a dinner that, although not large, was unfortunately high in fat. Susan was a superb gourmet cook and loved to entertain friends with her creamy culinary creativity.

Exercise didn't seem to help. She got up a half hour early every day to do some weight lifting with her husband in his home gym. "I'm so huge, I'd be embarrassed to go to aerobic classes," she lamented. She smoked one pack of cigarettes a day.

According to my calculations, if Susan got down to 161 pounds, she would be 22 percent fat. "You've got to be kidding!" she exclaimed. "I'd still be a blimp at that weight! When I weighed 145, I looked really good." I didn't argue with her. Chances were she had added quite a bit of lean muscle to lug around all that fat. I expected her to lose some of that muscle, but I was going to do everything I could to make sure she lost as little as possible. I wanted Susan to get down to 172 pounds in six months, a loss of 24 pounds, or 1 pound a week. Safe *fat loss* is usually limited to 1 to 2 pounds a week. If you're losing more than that, you are probably shedding a lot of muscle and water along with the fat. I wanted to make changes in Susan's eating and exercise habits without causing too great a disruption in her lifestyle. So I whipped out a poster of the Target Diet and told her that for the next six months, she could only eat from the center of the Target. To a gourmet cook, that's a pretty dramatic change! But I appealed to her creative nature. "Hey! Anyone can make things taste good if they add enough butter and cream. Let's see you do it with herbs and spices."

Susan was a sport and rose to the challenge. She bought every low-fat cookbook in her local bookstore, gathered up willing hungry friends, and became the best fatless cook around. She's even in the process of writing her own collection of recipes.

She needed to break the one-meal-a-day habit, which encourages fat storage (see the chapter "Diet"). We added a cereal and fruit breakfast. She didn't have time to go out for a regular lunch but agreed to have a minimum of four fruit or vegetable snacks throughout the day. Her daily calorie intake was around 1800.

Her evening drink before dinner was just a way of relaxing after work. We calculated that the drink added 100 calories, while a half hour on a stationary bicycle would burn up 100 calories. When she substituted one for the other, she got a 200-calorie deficit and actually felt *more* relaxed. "After sweating thirty minutes with Dan Rather, I'm ready for anything!"

When a woman is over 32 percent fat, I want her to spend a lot of time doing mild exercise. Four to six fifteen-minute sessions a day would be ideal. Since Susan worked, we couldn't fit this into her schedule. So instead we had her do two thirty-minute sessions a day with one day off a week. ("Monday! I hate Mondays.") One session was her evening martini substitute. The other session was in the morning when she usually lifted weights with her husband. We changed that because of time constraints. I didn't think Susan was motivated enough to do aerobics *plus* weight lifting, and aerobics is far superior for weight loss. As a replacement, Susan exercised to videotapes on her VCR. This worked well on the mornings she had to work and didn't want to go outdoors. She bought a variety of easy, low-impact programs, donned her sexiest leotard, and let loose without fear of giggles from onlookers. On weekends she briskly walked around the neighborhood with her husband. She was thus able to spend a lot of time exercising, and the diversity of activities actually seemed to improve her knee.

Her biggest problem was giving up smoking. Quitting the habit was tough. "I cut up carrots into little cigarette-sized sticks and stuffed them into empty cigarette packs. Then, whenever I got the urge, I slowly munched on one of the sticks. They sort of have a little nicotine flavor from being in the pack. Weird, but it worked." But weight gain is almost inevitable when you stop smoking. And sure enough, in spite of the other changes we instituted, Susan didn't lose a pound for three weeks. Luckily she

Smoking and Weight Gain

You've heard it often. "If I quit smoking I'll gain weight!" Most of us think that the weight gain is caused by the "munchies," the dreaded overeating that strikes former smokers.

Research shows that "it ain't necessarily so." Body fat tests were done on three groups of former smokers:

- The control group ate what they wanted.
- The second group carefully watched diet and did not eat more food.
- The third group did not eat more AND added daily exercise.

As expected, those in the first group gained weight. But surprisingly, the other two groups gained weight also! The second group gained about half as much as the first, and the third group gained about a third as much. What's going on?!!

Unhappy as it may make you, the weight gain is actually a sign that your body is getting healthier. Everyone knows that cigarettes are bad for the lungs. But they are also bad for your intestines. Smoke makes your intestinal lining so raw and irritated that many nutrients that would normally be absorbed are allowed to pass through. Say you eat a Twinkie. "Oh, hell," your beleaguered intestine groans, "let it go through!" When you stop smoking, the intestinal lining becomes pink and healthy again. Nutrients that once were wasted are now absorbed and you gain weight. Yes, it's discouraging, but if you watch your diet and exercise as the third group did, then the gain should be minimal (two to five pounds) and temporary. A few extra pounds is worth the years — more active, fun years — you'll add to your life.

didn't gain weight either. So we figured she was only three pounds behind schedule. And she was feeling great! "Every other time I tried to quit smoking, I've been a bear! But all this exercising and learning new recipes has taken my mind off it."

When six months were up, Susan went to her physician. I'd love to tell you that the exercise was so beneficial that she no longer needed the surgery, but that would be a fairy-tale ending. I *can* tell you that she recovered from the surgery much faster than her doctor expected and was back exercising her usual half-hour in the morning and in the evening after two months. For the surgery, she got down to 168 pounds and 30 percent fat, which means that of the 28 pounds she lost, 20 were fat and 8 were lean. I wasn't worried about the 8 pounds. I knew that about half of it was water and half was the extra muscle needed to carry unnecessary fat. In contrast, rapid weight loss diets have ratios of one to one — for every pound of fat lost, a pound of muscle goes with it.

Susan lost 1 percent fat per month, which is more than I recommend, but when the fat is high to begin with, this kind of drop sometimes occurs. By the end of the year, she was down to 160 pounds and 27 percent fat, which means she lost 7 more pounds of fat and 1 more pound of lean. To many of my female readers, her weight still may seem awfully high. But Susan is a big woman. Her lean body mass is 117 pounds. She has more bone and muscle weight than the *total* weight of some of her smaller friends. At 160 pounds she looks shapely because her fat is relatively low. Another woman, with the same weight but a lower lean body mass, would just look fat. Our goal for her is 152 pounds and 23 percent fat. I know she can do it. Her leaner friends — the lucky recipients of her new low-fat gourmet cooking — and Dan Rather agree.

Heart Rate As an Indicator of Exercise

YOU HAVE at your fingertips a marvelous device for testing your exercise program — your heart rate. For nearly everyone, one of the first parameters to change when you improve your physical condition is heart rate. As you become more and more fit, your resting pulse drops lower and lower. Very fit athletes sometimes have resting heart rates as low as 40 beats per minute. Even the moderate exerciser can expect her resting heart rate to drop 5 to 10 beats per minute.

A rise in heart rate can be a first warning that your body is overtrained or stressed. Triathletes and ultra-long-distance runners feel that if their morning heart rate jumps by 10 beats per minute, their body is overtrained; if they don't let up, they'll do worse, not better, in the race. As much as forty-eight hours before the onset of cold or flu symptoms, some people notice an elevated heart rate. They may feel fine, but their bodies are giving early signals that all is not right. To sum up, your *resting* heart rate slows down as you get fitter. It speeds up when your fitness is impaired, either through overtraining or sickness.

Your *exercise* heart rate is also a wonderful fitness measuring tool. By maintaining a pulse that is between 65 and 80 percent of maximum while you are exercising, you can be sure of reaping the greatest aerobic benefits. At this rate you burn the most fat, and your body is most likely to undergo all the other changes I discussed in earlier chapters.

Feedback from readers of *Fit or Fat?* indicates that there is a big problem with monitoring exercise through heart rate. Apparently, people are relying too much on the heart rate tables. For aerobic benefits, your heart rate during exercise shouldn't exceed 80 percent of your maximum heart rate. The problem arises in trying to determine your maximum. Generally speaking, maximum heart rate decreases with age. In about 86 percent of people the maximum can be determined simply by subtracting age from 220. If you are 35, your maximum heart rate would be 220 − 35 = 185. This formula is so well established that it can be found in lay press articles as well as the scientific literature where it originated. It is given in *Fit or Fat?* along with a table of maximum heart rates and recommended exercise heart rates.

However, about 7 percent of people are born with small hearts. To compensate for their small size these hearts have high maximum rates. Another 7 percent are the opposite — they have large hearts that "max out" at a lower rate than would be expected for their age. I don't want to imply that these people's hearts are ill or malfunctioning or pathologic; they are just different from the majority. If you are thirty-five years old, your maximum, according to the standard formula, should be 185. But say you go for a hard run, take what you feel is close to your maximum heart rate, and get 200. You try again three days in a row with similar results. You aren't sick; you just have a higher than average heart rate. Aerobic exercise for you would be 80 percent of 200 rather than 80 percent of 185.

We see plenty of examples of the opposite — people who can't get their heart rate up to the predicted levels. In fact, I belong to the latter category myself. My predicted maximum heart rate is 165, but my heart won't go over 155 no matter how fast I run or how hard I bicycle. So I'm getting good aerobic exercise when I jog at 80 percent of 155 = 124.

If you are nervous (for obvious reasons) about running at maximum to determine your maximum heart rate, and you don't want to have a stress test done on a treadmill, then you won't know your true (actual) maximum heart rate. You must then use the standard formula for an approximation.

Actually, if I could run alongside you, I could identify your aerobic exercise level quite accurately simply by observation. Your degree of breathlessness while jogging for a sustained fifteen to twenty minutes is a better indicator of aerobic level than pulse. If I were running with you, I might ask, "Where are you from?" If you gasp out a one-word answer, "Ohio," I would tell you to slow down. On the other hand, if you rattle off, "I'm from Canton, Ohio. I live on West 63rd in a split-level, four-bedroom, two-thousand-square-foot home with my husband, three kids, dog, and a parakeet," I would ask you to run faster. Ideally, an aerobic pace allows the person to speak in short, halting phrases: "I'm from Ohio — (pant, pant) — near the outskirts of Toledo — (pant, pant) — in a little farming community."

Too often, well-meaning aerobic instructors or gym personnel are sticklers when it comes to heart rate. They admonish their clients to speed up or slow down so that their heartbeats per min-

---

The incidence of heart attack during exercise is so low that when one does occur it is reported in the newspapers. In contrast, heart attacks in sedentary individuals are so common as to be a national disgrace. It becomes obvious that a sedentary life is far more dangerous than an athletic life. To insist on a stress electrocardiogram before undertaking an exercise program misses the point. Instead, perhaps we should take a stress electrocardiogram if we plan *not* to exercise, because if we are not in perfect physical condition, a sedentary lifestyle may kill us.

ute match a chart on a wall. They ignore patterns of breathing or comments such as, "This is sure hard!" (or "too easy!") Studies at various exercise testing laboratories have shown that simply *asking* a person how hard he is working is a more reliable indicator than heart rate. Researchers call this the "perceived rate of exertion." Most people can settle on a good aerobic exercise level for themselves if they are left alone.

One person, obsessed with the idea that heart rate was the *only* criterion for measuring exercise, invented a sauna that blew hot air, which causes the heart rate to increase. He thought that all he would have to do was sit in the sauna with a pulsemeter strapped to his chest. An operator would control the heat until the participant's pulse came up to his training heart rate. He would sit in this hot little hurricane for twenty minutes reading *Playboy* while his body became physically fit. We laugh at this scheme because we know that getting fit is more than just a matter of passively increasing heart rate. Muscles need to be exercised, the lungs must be worked, there has to be *activity*. As I discussed earlier, manipulating the symptom only (taking antihistamines for cold symptoms, dieting for overfat problems) does not correct the systemic disorder. To get a systemic response, you need to do whole-body, systemic exercise.

Heart rate can tell you many things. It lets you know if you're getting fitter, and it lets you know if you're *not* getting fitter. It tells you when you're exercising too hard or not hard enough. But it's only a tool. Use heart rate formulas as a back-up to your own common sense, not as the only indicators of exercise level, ignoring other signals the body is sending. I put the heart formulas in *Fit or Fat?* because they are useful, but they are not as accurate as I would like.

No Pain, No Gain?

A WOMAN ONCE COMPLAINED to me, "When I do my exercise class, the instructor keeps pushing me to work harder — no pain, no gain. But you tell me to slow down. Who's right?" The answer is, we both are right! How hard or gently you should exercise depends on what you're trying to accomplish. If you want to lose fat, go easy. If you want to build muscle, you need to work hard.

Any time a small muscle is made to lift a heavy weight, especially if several repetitions are required, a sharp burning pain is felt in the muscle. The pain is caused by lactic acid, which indicates that the exercise is *an*aerobic, meaning without oxygen. When you weight lift, the muscle tissue swells, causing pressure on the blood vessels around it. The flow of blood to the muscle is lessened, and therefore less oxygen is supplied. When oxygen is limited, muscle metabolism is hindered, glucose is only partially metabolized, and lactic acid is produced. The build-up of lactic acid in a muscle is painful but temporary. When the exercise ceases, blood rushes in and the pain goes away.

Good examples of this phenomenon abound. Sit-ups, for example, demand that the very thin abdominal muscles lift the entire upper body: head, shoulders, arms, and chest. If all the abdominal muscles of a large, strong man were cut away, you could easily hold them in one hand. Now imagine that man's upper body in your other hand, and you understand my phrase, "a small muscle lifting a large weight." Typical weight lifting exercises are of this type, making each muscle, or group of muscles, lift so much weight that ten or twelve repetitions totally fatigue the muscles and produce lactic acid pain.

If you think about it, you'll realize that many calisthenic exercises are really a form of weight lifting. A sit-up uses the upper body as a weight instead of iron plates. Push-ups also make use of upper-body weight instead of barbells or dumbbells. As I mention various exercises, notice the ratio of amount of muscle used to amount of weight used. Sit-ups use a relatively small amount of muscle for the weight lifted so that abdominal fatigue occurs quickly and lactic acid is produced quickly. Men are typically larger in the chest and shoulders than women, so sit-ups are even harder for them. Push-ups, on the other hand, use a bit more muscle compared to weight, so some people can do them for hours. Side leg lifts are done with the abductor muscle, which is only a small fraction of the muscle on the thigh. People are often fooled by this exercise, believing that the entire thigh muscle is doing the work. The abductor is quite small, and the leg may be quite large. Leg lifts produce lactic acid in the abductor quickly.

The expression "weight lifting" means lifting a heavy weight with a small muscle; it means quick fatigue and soreness; and it means lactic acid. The definition does not extend to the use of two- and four-pound hand weights. Even carrying seventy pounds in a backpack doesn't produce lactic acid and isn't called weight lifting. For the sake of clarity, "weight lifting" is defined only as (1) heavy-weight, (2) anaerobic, (3) lactic-acid-producing exercise that enhances the size and hardness of muscle but *does not burn fat*.

The muscle pain caused by lactic acid, called the "burn," is believed by many people to be necessary for maximum muscle growth. In fact, body builders deliberately induce the burn to achieve the greatest bulk and definition of muscle.

Let me stress that lactic acid pain is produced by *anaerobic* exercise. *Aerobic* (fat-burning) exercise is not painful! With aerobic exercise the slogan should be, "No pain, maintain." Or, better yet, "No pain, fat wanes." The no pain, no gain theory applies to muscle *growth* and is anaerobic. The amount of protein in muscle increases when the muscle is subjected to repeated oxygen deficits. It says, "What if she keeps doing this? I've got to get stronger!"

No pain, no gain does *not* lead to fat loss! Muscle burn indicates increased *glucose* expenditure, not fat expenditure. So, if you've got fat thighs and you're pushing yourself to do 200 leg lifts, thinking, "Oh boy, I must really be burning up my fat!" you're wrong! You're just going to end up with big, strong, *and* fat legs. Your best approach is to mix aerobic exercise for fat loss with intense, lactic-acid-producing exercises to make the muscles in your legs more shapely.

Slow Exercise Burns Off
More Fat Than Intense Exercise

THERE'S A FAT MAN on my jogging route. Every time I see him, he's running as fast as he can, panting and wheezing, his face as red as a beet. I once asked him, "Why do you run so fast?" Looking at me as if I had a double-digit IQ, he haughtily replied, "To burn more calories, of course, and get rid of this fat!" He was doing everything wrong — and was stubborn about learning something new. If that description fits the man in your life, please read this chapter to him.

It's true that the faster you run, the more calories your body uses. The problem is that burning lots of calories isn't the same as burning lots of fat. Muscles use fat *and* carbohydrates to produce energy. However, when muscles are pushed to high exercise levels, they use mostly blood glucose for metabolism and rely very little on fat. So the faster you exercise, the more blood sugar and stored sugar you burn, but very little fat.

We used to assume that after intense exercise, we would lose fat as the body converted it into sugar to replace what was just lost. But research has shown that humans don't have the internal chemistry to convert fat into sugar. Fat doesn't break down to replace glucose. In fact, we can't convert fat into anything. The shocking conclusion is that fat is lost ONLY ONLY ONLY by burning it in the muscle during moderate to slow exercise. When we exercise very hard, anaerobically, we just burn sugar and hardly any fat at all.

Pretend that you are out of shape so that you can't jog comfortably with the average jogger. For you, let's say, a twelve-minute-per-mile pace is maximum if you want to remain aerobic, not breathless. This would be the fastest you could go and still expect to burn off some fat. One day, as you jog along at your comfortable fat-burning pace, another woman zooms past you at a nine-minute pace. The other woman may appear to be fatter than you; in fact, she may *be* fatter than you. So you assume that she is running too fast, isn't burning any fat, and hasn't read this chapter. This could be true. But it could also be that she has very fit muscles underneath the exterior fat so that her nine-minute pace is as fat-burning for her as your twelve-minute pace is for you. Perhaps she was once much fatter than you, so she still has some fat to lose even though she's fitter underneath. If you speed up to run with her, you will run breathlessly and burn almost no fat at all.

I'm not saying that people should never run fast and never do sprints. Athletes use such anaerobic exercise for special reasons. But even the athlete must include slow, long-distance exercise to keep body fat down. It sounds odd, but the only way to speed up the fat-burning adaptation is to spend more time exercising slowly and gently. To speed it up, you've got to slow it down.

Alice

WHEN ALICE WAS FORTY years old she was forty pounds overweight. Her friends threw her an over-the-hill birthday party complete with black armbands and black balloons. But Alice was a
cheerful woman. Reaching "middle age" didn't bother her, and
besides, her friends also brought lots of barbecued spareribs,
French fries, creamy coleslaw, and scrumptious, gooey desserts.
Alice went to bed that night feeling great about her friends and life
in general. At 2 A.M. she woke up with nausea and an acute pain
in her upper right side. The next day her doctor took one look at
the plump, blond woman and said, "Hmph! Fair, fat, and forty!
You may have gallbladder problems." He put her on a high-carbohydrate, low-fat, low-calorie diet. Over the next two years she
gradually lost thirty pounds. If she weakened now and then, suc-
cumbing to one too many chocolate chip cookies, her "body-
guard," the gallbladder, was painfully sure to let her know.

Alice started feeling so much better that she took up exercise to
lose the last ten pounds. She had tried jogging when she was quite
overweight, but it was just too much. With her new, slimmer
body, she was ready to try something new. And who would be a
better coach than her husband, who had always been involved in
sports? The first day he decided that calisthenics were in order, so
they did jumping jacks, push-ups, twists, turns, whatever. Alice

was so exhausted that on the last twenty jumping straddles she landed too hard on one leg, twisting her ankle. That put her out of commission for about a month.

When she was ready to try again, David said, "Honey, you're just not coordinated enough to do the calisthenics. We're going to run every day, and don't worry, I'll slow my pace down for you." David is six foot two. For Alice, five foot five and out of condition, he slowed his pace all the way down to an eight-minute mile.

Amazingly, Alice stuck to his program for three weeks, bravely staggering along, gasping for air. She developed shin splints, and the pain, along with her constant exhaustion, got the best of her usually cheerful nature.

One morning at breakfast, she confessed, "David, I just can't keep up with those long legs of yours."

"Don't be silly," Dave said with a smile. "Foxes run just as fast as giraffes. Cheetahs have been clocked at seventy miles an hour. You're just lazy about exercise."

"Well, what do I do to get beyond this awful fatigue? Honestly, I feel trashed the whole rest of the day!"

"You've just got to keep pushing. Look at me. I've been doing it all my life. I wouldn't have been all-star in college football if I had taken a day off because I felt lazy. Now, come on, get your running shoes on. Today, we're going twice as far. You'll thank me for it in the end."

Alice's reply is unprintable. Good old Dave ran by himself that morning.

Later that day, Alice ran into an old friend. When the friend asked if she had been ill, she looked so drawn and tired, Alice burst into tears. "I'm so miserable! I just wish I were fat again!" Alice and her friend talked for quite a while.

"Alice, I don't think David realizes how hard exercise is for you because it comes so easily to him. The sad thing is that the harder a beginner pushes, the *less* likely she is to improve. I'm a marathon runner and in good condition, but even I benefited from slowing down. For a long time, I kept testing at 18 percent fat. I really wanted to be 14 percent, but no matter how hard I trained, I couldn't get my fat down. Finally, the people who were testing me suggested I *slow down*. That didn't make much sense to me, but they said the body responds to gentle pressure. So I thought, what the heck, going slower for a while would be a welcome break. It was uncanny! In six months my fat went right down to 14 percent!"

So Alice suggested to David that they run separately for a while. He was glad to get back to his faster pace without an irritable wife trailing behind. Alice switched to a comfortable eleven-minute mile. Soon she really looked forward to her daily jaunt. Her good humor returned, and the marriage was saved! She also lost that last ten pounds.

There's nothing unique about Alice's story. She didn't go on to become the neighborhood running celebrity. Her method for weight loss wasn't spectacular — just practical. She learned how to lose weight and keep it off by dieting sensibly and exercising slowly. No, her story won't make the newspaper headlines. But it should.

Spot Reducing and Cellulite

As far as I know, other than surgery, there is no way to spot-reduce; that is, it is impossible to lose fat selectively from a particular area of the body. As the saying goes, "If spot reducing worked, people who chew gum would have skinny faces." Nonetheless, the desire to "fix" a bulging fatty place is so strong that a million gimmicks are available for the gullible to try:

Saunas, steam baths
Body wraps, herbal wraps
Rollers, fanny bumpers

Tummy belts, tummy
    tightener wheels
Fancy weight systems
Exercising in plastic suits

One of the most inventive rip-offs I've heard about is the idea of using a home vacuum cleaner to suck fat from the body. A kit was sold as a special attachment which led from the vacuum cleaner to a pair of loose-fitting pants with drawstrings at the waist and knees. Various exercises had to be done, presumably to loosen up the fat, so that when the vacuum was turned on, presto! all was sucked away. I wonder if instructions were included on how to remove all that fat from inside the vacuum cleaner.

Spot-reducing devices, gimmicks, and exercises don't work! They don't work because fat, no matter where it is located, belongs to your whole body, not just to the muscles in one place. Fat is part of your bank of calories, which is drawn upon when you exercise aerobically. It's easy to see why people get tied into the idea of spot reducing. After all, hair can be removed from a specific area and muscles can be built in specific areas. Women can change so many specific things in specific areas, like mascara on eyes, polish on fingernails, that it's easy to think fat can be removed from a specific area. But fat isn't like that; it's like blood. If you slash your wrist, you don't get wrist blood — you get blood. The fat on your thighs isn't thigh fat — it's fat. The fat on your tummy isn't tummy fat — it's fat. A doctor would say of any pocket of fat, "It's systemic." The blood in your finger doesn't belong to your finger. It moves in and out. The fat in your thigh doesn't belong to your thigh. Like blood, it continuously moves in and out of an area so that it is available anywhere for aerobic use. When you do an aerobic exercise, such as running, your leg muscle doesn't say, "Send me some leg fat." It says, "Send me some fat — any kind, from anywhere."

Fat cannot be rubbed off. It can't be melted away. When you think about it, spot reducing really is silly. You don't see very fit athletes worrying about little spots of fat here and there. They've earned their trim bodies the hard way. They worked at it. The *only* way to get rid of fat, short of surgery, is to work it off with aerobic exercise.

You may argue that spot reducing works because you've been doing leg raises for years, and now your legs appear to be much slimmer. Actually, the leg raises made the *muscles* in your legs firmer so that the area looks less fat. An increase in muscle protein has occurred rather than a decrease in fat. Exercises for specific parts of the body are excellent for firming and shaping the underlying muscle and hence reshaping the body, but you must do systemic, whole-body exercise (preferably on your feet) to remove fat, no matter where it is.

The popularity of aerobic exercise classes makes these facts particularly pertinent. You might attend such a program and find that most of the class time is spent on exercises for specific muscles, such as leg lifts and sit-ups. Such a class would be largely nonaerobic, despite its name. Anytime you are on the floor, you are not doing aerobics and therefore not accomplishing a lot of fat reduction. The only aerobic part of such classes is when you are on your feet, jumping, weaving, dodging, dancing — call it what you will — but to be aerobic it must gently warm up your whole body rather than tire one muscle group. The better aerobic instructors keep students on their feet for at least twenty minutes of continuous exercise to decrease fat and then work on individual muscle groups for toning and firming. The kinds of exercises that produce the so-called burn should really be termed spot-*building* exercises rather than spot-reducing ones. They enhance body shape by emphasizing a particular area, thus making surrounding areas appear slimmer. You *can* spot build. You *cannot* spot reduce.

Be aware that your legs may get bigger in the first months of aerobics. The leg muscles enlarge while little, if any, leg fat is lost because most of the fat loss is occurring in the upper body. You may get discouraged as your thighs get larger and your upper body gets smaller. Only when total body fat approaches 22 percent do the legs start to lose fat and get smaller. Many women's legs stay the same for two or more years, even on the best of exercise/diet programs. Such apparent setbacks make women quite susceptible to quack exercise schemes and quick weight loss diets.

Cellulite is just plain old fat deposited in areas where the skin and underlying support tissue tend to pucker and wrinkle. It isn't a special kind of fat but rather a special kind of skin over the fat. After all, we tend to grow hair in some places more than others and form calluses in some places more easily than in others. It's not hard to imagine that certain areas of skin are more susceptible than others to sagging or pocketing from underlying fat. Some women, regardless of their percent of fat, are more prone to showing subcutaneous fat than others for the same reason that some women have more hair than others. In general, fair-skinned women seem to have more puckering, or cellulite, than darker, thicker-skinned women. In a similar manner, some women get extreme stretch marks delivering small babies, while their sisters get few or no stretch marks delivering large babies.

In the end, cellulite is just a descriptive word for an area on the body where fat and skin take on a particular appearance. There is nothing particularly different about its chemistry. Since cellulite is typically found on the lower body, you aren't likely to see any decrease in it if you are over 22 percent total fat. There are surgical techniques for fat removal in cellulite areas, but surgeons are quick to admit that this does not always correct the puckering problem. In some cases, the removal of underlying fat tissue actually augments the rippling of the overlying skin. Surgeons hesitate to try it on obviously fat people because the cellulite areas may look worse instead of better. Women who still have cellulite after reducing their total body fat to less than 22 percent via exercise and diet are the best candidates for surgical removal.

Diet

WHY IN THE WORLD do people continue to think potatoes are fattening? And bread? And most other carbohydrates? I don't know how these beliefs started, but they're wrong! A medium baked potato has 100 calories. That's not a lot of calories. The problem is what you add to it. Two pats of butter and a little sour cream add enough fat to the potato to make it 250 calories. Only 100 calories, or 40 percent of all that, is really food. Look at it this way; over half of the calories in that mess are pure grease, devoid of vitamins, minerals, or protein.

Let's say it again. POTATOES ARE NOT FATTENING! Neither is bread or pasta or other "starchy" foods. Why do such foolish notions persist? IT'S FAT THAT IS FATTENING. The amount of calories in fat is quite astonishing. Eight almonds, because they are so high in fat, have as many calories as a huge baked potato. A small hamburger patty can have as many calories as an overflowing cup of beans. One quarter-pound stick of butter equals fifteen slices of whole wheat bread. Just visualize the difference in size in these examples. Very small fatty foods can be replaced by much larger, more filling, and more satisfying carbohydrate foods.

I've said it over and over — get the fat out of your diet.

Fatty foods are tremendously concentrated so that a very small amount gives a surprising number of calories. On airplane trips, you push away 60 calories of rice or potatoes on your plate but

The Covert Bailey Guarantee:

If you get the fat out of your diet, I promise that you will get the fat out of your body.

think nothing of eating the small package of peanuts worth 90 calories.

The trick is to know how much fat is in a food. Even if you do a lot of cooking and are aware of the fat in foods, it is easy to be fooled by labels. Did you realize that 2 percent fat milk is actually 30 percent fat calories? In other words, fat is only 2 percent of the milk by weight, but it contributes 30 percent of the calories. A gram of fat, which is about the size of a bouillon cube, contains 9 calories, while the same amount of carbohydrate contains only 4 calories. This one little bit of information allows you to get around the misleading sales hype on food labels.

You may be conned into buying a high-fat or high-sugar product because of a taste-tempting picture or healthful-sounding name. Words like "pure," "natural," and "unrefined" are sure sellers these days. But you should know that the name on the label can be practically anything the manufacturer chooses because it's considered a title. However, the box of nutrition information on the back of the container is strictly controlled by the Food and Drug Administration (FDA). The listing must be accurate, have a particular sequence, and leave nothing out. All you have to do is look at the number of calories per serving and then compare that with the number of calories coming from fat (which is the number of grams of fat times 9). I believe that a diet with a total of 30 percent calories from fat is pretty good. Twenty percent would be better. The Pritikin Diet pushes 10 percent. The diet of the average American is 50 percent fat calories, which, coupled with no exercise, is why we are so fat.

For practice, try this. Suppose you don't want to cook dinner, so you and your husband go to the store to buy a frozen dinner.

Veal parmigiana sounds good to both of you. He selects Stouffer's Dinner Supreme Veal Parmigiana with pasta Alfredo and with green beans and red peppers seasoned with butter sauce. Armour Dinner Classics Veal Parmigiana looks more appealing to you, with its Italian-style mixed vegetables and spaghetti with garlic butter sauce. Let's analyze both dinners to see who made the better selection.

	Stouffer's Dinner Supreme	*Armour Dinner Classics*
Serving size:	12.25 ounces	10.75 ounces
Total calories:	370	430
Fat:	15 grams	25 grams
Fat calories:	$15 \times 9 = 135$	$25 \times 9 = 225$
% of calories from fat:	$135/370 = 36\%$	$225/430 = 52\%$

Your husband's selection provides more food in spite of containing fewer calories and also fewer fat calories.

Here are two more labels from frozen meals:

	Product A	*Product B**
Serving size:	6.5 ounces	6.5 ounces
Total calories:	270	355
Fat:	16 grams	16 grams
Fat calories:	144	144
% of calories from fat:	53%	41%

*Actual product weight is 10.25 ounces. I used 6.5 ounces of the product, adjusting the other numbers accordingly so that the two products could be easily compared.

Not much difference between the two, is there? Product A is Weight Watchers Southern Fried Chicken Patty, while Product B is Swanson's Fried Chicken (White Portions) Dinner.

Don't let low-calorie products fool you. They are often quite high in fat. In a survey of my supermarket, I found that many frozen meals claiming to be ideal for someone watching her weight were 40–60 percent fat! True, *total* calories in these products are low, but it's because the quantity of food in the package is low. In other words, they aren't really low calorie, they are

> Eat, drink, but be wary,
> for tomorrow you may live.

low quantity. I believe women would fare better in lowering their body fat if they would concentrate on the percentage of fat in their foods rather than on the calories. Diet shouldn't mean deprivation. Fill up on carbohydrates, not fat. You will be less hungry (and, therefore, less likely to cheat on your diet) after a 500-calorie high-carbohydrate, low-fat meal than on a 500-calorie high-fat meal simply because there is more food in the low-fat meal to fill you up.

Get in the habit of routinely "guesstimating" the fat calories of products. It's not hard once you've tried it a few times. Sometimes a manufacturer doesn't provide a breakdown of calories or nutrients. By law they are required only to list ingredients. However, if the food claims to be "low calorie" or "reduced calorie," the manufacturer is required to give the nutrient breakdown. Reduced-calorie salad dressings, for example, always let you know how few calories they have compared to regular salad dressings. But you'll seldom find calorie content on a bottle of regular salad dressing.

If the nutrient breakdown is not printed on the label, then you have to rely on the list after the word "ingredients." These are listed in order of decreasing amount in the product. If fat or sugar is among the first four or five ingredients, it is not a low-calorie product.

Diet is incredibly simple. It's not the big complicated mess everyone wants to make of it. In fact, all you need to do is follow these four basic rules:

1. Eat less fat.
2. Eat less sugar.
3. Eat more fiber.
4. Eat a balanced diet.

When I was first writing this chapter, I considered including sections for people with "special requirements." There would be diet recommendations for the recovering anorexic or for the female body builder or for the postmenopausal woman. But when I started writing the various "prescriptions," I found that I was saying the same thing over and over: "Eat a balanced, low-fat, low-sugar, high-fiber diet." Calorie needs and vitamin/mineral requirements may fluctuate, but the basic recommendations remain the same.

The sad thing is that too many people ignore the basics in the search for the esoteric. They argue that advice about balanced, low-fat, low-sugar, high-fiber eating is old-fashioned, behind the times. They want to know about the additives and preservatives in foods. They're worried about saturated fats and cholesterol. But where do you find additives, preservatives, saturated fats, and cholesterol? They're in the high-fat, high-sugar foods! By sticking to the basic rules, you don't have to worry about them.

A bit more complicated is the concern people have about vitamins and minerals. Most people's vitamin and mineral requirements are met by following the four basic rules outlined above. When there is less fat in meals, the volume of food consumed can be safely increased without increasing calories. If more food is eaten, vitamin/mineral needs are more likely to be satisfied and even exceeded.

For instance, women worry about getting enough calcium. By switching from whole milk to skim milk and drinking twice as much, they can double their calcium intake yet have no increase in calories. Three glasses of skim milk add up to 270 calories, no fat, and all the calcium a woman needs for the day. Unfortunately, many women cut out milk altogether, calling it "baby food," and eat cheeses for their calcium needs. Most cheeses are 70–80 percent fat. You can satisfy your calcium needs by eating 5 ounces of cheese every day, but you'll be getting 575 calories, of which 400 are fat calories. Moreover, 5 ounces of cheese isn't very much volume. You will feel more filled up with three glasses of skim milk, even though the milk has fewer calories.

Vitamin and mineral deficiencies occur when your diet is unbalanced or too low in calories. Who is the most likely candidate for low-calorie, unbalanced dieting? The overfat woman. Active women need about 2000 calories a day. By eating from all four food groups and restricting fat, a woman eating 2000 calories a day can easily fulfill her vitamin and mineral requirements. But when calories are reduced, vitamin and mineral needs may be more difficult to satisfy. If she gets only 1000 to 1400 calories a day, there is a possibility that vitamin needs *may not* be met. Careful attention to balancing the diet is essential. This is sometimes difficult, and it's *possible* that some vitamin or mineral is lacking. For people eating only 1000 calories per day, I recommend a vitamin/mineral supplement. It doesn't have to be anything fancy. I wish a manufacturer would market a pill that supplies 50 percent of the recommended daily allowance (RDA) instead of the usual 100 percent. After all, the food you eat, even if you don't eat much of it, does fulfill most of your vitamin and mineral requirements.

Two further basic rules for women:

5. Eat foods high in iron. The daily requirement is 18 milligrams (mg.).
6. Eat foods high in calcium. The daily requirement is 1000 mg.

In dietary studies, many, many women are found to be quite low in these two nutrients. Iron deficiency has been found in over 60 percent of all women. Women who rely on fruits and vegetables for their iron are sometimes surprised to discover they have iron deficiency anemia. Fruits and vegetables do have iron, but the body seems to handle better the iron found in red meat, one of the foods calorie-conscious women avoid. Calcium needs are also difficult to meet if a woman is watching her calories. Refer to the list of foods containing iron on page 60 and the calcium list at the end of "Fit Bones." If your diet is consistently low in either of these nutrients, then supplementation is in order.

And one final basic rule:

7. The fatter you are, the *more often* you should eat.

Studies of rats have shown that fasting or eating one meal a day actually encourages the storage of fat. The body panics when food isn't provided on a regular basis and tends to "save" calories by storing them as fat. If 1200 calories a day are spread out over five or six small meals, fewer of them will be stored as fat than if all of the 1200 calories are consumed at one time.

The chart below gives you guidelines on how much fat should be in your diet. Get one of the many fat gram counters available to determine how much fat you are eating. Then, depending on how fat you are and how much fat you need to lose, modify your meals so that you are eating a 25 percent, 20 percent, or 10 percent fat diet. (For more specific information on low-fat cooking, refer to *The Fit-or-Fat Target Diet* and *Target Recipes*.)

The most obvious result of poor nutrition in America today is obesity. I didn't call this book *Women and Their Iron* or *Women and Their Vitamin Requirements*, because these problems are mi-

Recommended Daily Calories and Grams of Fat for Women

	If your percentage of body fat is:	If you don't know your percentage of body fat, but you:	You should eat: Calories/day	You should eat: Grams of fat/ day
25% fat diet	22% fat or less	are satisfied with your present weight	1700–2000	55
20% fat diet	23–35%	want to lose 5–15 lbs.	1400–1700	30–40
10% fat diet	36% fat or more	want to lose more than 15 lbs.	1000–1400	10–15

Iron Content of Foods

1–1.5 mg.

Custard, 1 cup
Pudding, 1 cup
Egg, 1 whole
Crabmeat, 1 cup
Most fish, 3 oz.
Lamb, 3 oz.
Chicken, 3 oz.
Apple, grapefruit, grape,
    cranberry juice, 1 cup
Avocado, 1
Banana, 1
Blackberries, blueberries,
    raspberries, strawberries,
    1 cup
Cantaloupe, 1 half
Peaches, 2 whole
Rhubarb, 1 cup
Most breads, 1 slice
Cereal, 1 cup
Macaroni, noodles, pasta, rice,
    1 cup
Most non–dark green vegetables,
    1 cup

2–2.5 mg.

Sardines, 3 oz.
Shrimp, 3 oz.
Tuna, 3 oz.
Pork, 3 oz.
Dates, 10 whole
Prunes, 6 large
Raisins, ½ cup
Most nuts, ½ cup
Spinach, ½ cup cooked
Dark green vegetables, 1 cup
    cooked

3–3.5 mg.

Clams, 3 oz.
Beef and veal, 3 oz.
Blackstrap molasses, 1 tbsp.

4–5 mg.

Most iron-supplemented cereals,
    1 cup
Most dried beans, 1 cup cooked
Beef heart, 3 oz.

6–7 mg.

Liver, 3 oz.
Dried apricots and peaches,
    1 cup

nor compared to the problems associated with obesity. When you
visit Uncle Joe in the hospital he's probably not there because of
malnutrition or a vitamin deficiency. He's there because he has
some fat-related disease such as heart attack, diabetes, or stroke.
I once knew a man who had installed a fancy camper atop his
little four-cylinder truck. He couldn't understand why the vehicle

was so underpowered and kept putting additives in the gas tank to speed it up. Some people do the same thing to their bodies. They tow around a trailer load of fat and then take vitamin and mineral supplements because they have "low energy." The American who worries about getting enough vitamins in the face of overwhelming obesity is comparable to a stark-naked man asking his wife, "Which belt should I wear today?"

Learn to eat a low-fat, low-sugar, high-fiber diet. Questions about vitamins, minerals, and the like become superfluous if your diet is well balanced and sufficient in calories.

Don't be ripped off by new diet scams. There are already too many diet books. Everyone is searching for inside information on the newest way to lose weight. Probably the number-one gimmick used to sell diet books is the promise of "quick weight loss," which is an automatic tip-off that it isn't genuine. You see, the fatter a person is, the less competent her body is at:

1. Releasing fat from fat cells
2. Preventing calories from entering fat cells
3. Burning fat for calories

As a result, the fatter you are, the less able you are to get rid of fat.

Picture some very full fat cells on your left hip. Each of those fat cells is an independent living organism that has stored its hoard of fat for a reason. You want the cells to release that fat, and you want your muscles to burn it up. If you are out of shape or fat, your fat cells don't release fat readily and your muscles don't burn it readily. No matter what you do, you won't lose fat quickly. Even very fit athletes can't burn off five pounds of fat in a week, yet many diet books claim a five-pound weight loss per week. Such claims are a clear sign of deceit, because the weight a fat person loses that quickly is mostly water weight. Some protein will be lost on such a diet and, finally, a pound of fat, at most.

The fatter and more out of shape a person is, the slower the fat loss becomes and the less colorful the claims on a book's cover should be. An honest weight loss book should proclaim, "Guaranteed no more than one pound per week weight loss." Or perhaps, "Guaranteed agonizingly slow weight loss."

In addition to claiming fast weight loss, the really flaky diets claim that their special combinations of foods and chemicals increase fat metabolism dramatically, causing fat cells to practically throw out their fat. Virtually every fad diet ever written makes such claims; wouldn't you think people would wise up?

So! Let's go back to losing body fat the honest way. It will be slow and boring, you won't have dramatic things to report to your friends, but you just might achieve the change in metabolism that prevents you from getting fat again.

Now That I'm Exercising, Do I Need More Vitamins?

WHEN I WAS A BOY, a friend thought it would be fun to have a water-drinking contest to see who could consume the most. I gave up after about ten glasses, but my friend kept going. He died the next day. Unusual? Yes. Impossible? No! It's been popular lately to drink great quantities of water before an endurance event. Studies have shown that hyperhydration *can* aid in keeping the athlete's body temperature down and preventing dehydration. However, some people have gone too far, resulting in coma and/or death from water overdose. Even water, a seemingly harmless, totally natural substance, can kill you if you drink too much.

Most people view vitamins and minerals the same way they do water, as inherently safe. Yet every year thousands of cases of vitamin poisoning are reported. How many more people are suffering unreported overdose side effects from their naive abuse of vitamins? It's ironic to me that these are the people who are most concerned with their health. They try to eat well and exercise regularly. They're the first to scorn those who smoke, drink alcohol, or take drugs. Yet vitamins, taken in pharmacological doses, act as drugs. These "do-gooders" are, in a sense, drug abusers!

Let's look at what I call the vicious "megatoxic" cycle of vitamin overdose. Mary takes extra vitamin C because she read that it will help prevent colds. But vitamin C interferes with the absorption of copper and iron and increases the need for vitamin E. So Mary takes more vitamin E, copper, and iron to compensate. Vitamin E interferes with vitamins A and K, so Mary increases her intake of these fat-soluble, stored vitamins. By doing so she risks hypercalcemia, deposits in soft tissue, irreversible kidney damage, heart/lung damage, and liver damage. Wait a minute! There's more. Too much vitamin E causes depression, fatigue, and flu-like symptoms. Yes, you saw it coming. Poor, tired, depressed Mary feels like she's coming down with a cold and completes the megatoxic cycle by taking more vitamin C.

Of course, in this example I'm talking about tremendous overdoses, and most people don't go that far. I'm hoping that pointing out the very obvious toxicity caused by megadoses will help you understand the possible problems with lesser dosages.

Recently I read more carefully than usual one of the popular body building magazines. I was pleased with what it said. Since the articles were written for the lay public, they didn't have the scientific approach of technical journals, but most of the information was accurate and reliable. Credible journalism is the norm in most popular magazines today. Unfortunately, much of the advertising that accompanies the articles is blatantly ridiculous. A responsible article on calcium, for example, may be followed by an advertisement pushing calcium supplements. The author of the article may suggest supplements in certain circumstances, but the advertisers would have you believe that *everyone* needs them.

Bear in mind that manufacturers have almost no restrictions as to what they can say in their advertisement. Other than the required "Advertisement" label in the corner, they have virtual carte blanche. Body-shaping formulas, carbohydrate energizers, fat-reducing pills are all given credibility with their before-and-after pictures. "True testimonials" claim that various vitamins and minerals can improve everything from brain power to sexual performance. The point I am trying to make is that advertising has made people believe that large doses of vitamin and mineral supplements are absolutely essential, while every responsible writer on the subject of nutrition says just the opposite. In all the fitness magazines the same advice is written a hundred different ways; namely, a well-balanced, low-fat/sugar, high-carbohydrate diet is the surest way to enhance performance. You don't need to take supplements if you learn to eat right!

What about the statement that heavy exercise increases the need for both vitamin B and zinc? Yes, this *is* true. High-level athletics does increase the need for thiamine (vitamin B_1). But to conclude that this vitamin should be supplemented is erroneous. The high-carbohydrate diet I recommend easily meets the additional vitamin B requirement.

High-intensity exercise also demands more zinc for protein synthesis and tissue repair. But zinc is plentiful in our recommended diet, and taking supplements in addition to the diet can easily produce an overdose. It's been shown that high zinc intake lowers the level of HDL (high-density lipoprotein) cholesterol — the kind that protects against heart disease. Endurance exercise elevates this "good" cholesterol. How silly to negate the effects of your hard work with a pill!

People think that if a vitamin is water soluble it goes right through harmlessly. This is not quite accurate. Toxicity can and *does* occur with water-soluble vitamins. For example, if you insist on taking extra thiamine because you exercise a lot, you'll probably go into that vicious cycle I mentioned earlier. Large intakes of thiamine not only cause anaphylactic shock but also interfere with the absorption of the other B vitamins. If you take more B vitamins to overcome this, you're courting liver damage, depressed secretion of gastric hydrochloric acid, sleep disturbances, nerve damage, irregular heartbeat, and diarrhea. And, if

U.S. Recommended Daily Allowances (U.S. RDA) for Women[a]

Age	Wt.	Ht.	Calories	Protein[b] (grams)	Calcium (mg)	Phosphorus (mg)	Iron (mg)	Vit. A (I.U.)	Thiamine (mg)	Riboflavin (mg)	Niacin (mg)	Vit. C (mg)
11–14	101	5'2"	2200	46	1200	1200	18	5000	1.5	1.7	20	60
15–18	120	5'4"	2100	46	1200	1200	18	5000	1.5	1.7	20	60
19–22	120	5'4"	2100	45	1000	1000	18	5000	1.5	1.7	20	60
23–50	120	5'4"	2000	45	1000	1000	18	5000	1.5	1.7	20	60
51+	120	5'4"	1800	45	1000	1000	10	5000	1.5	1.7	20	60
Pregnant			+300	+30	+400	+400	+18[c]	+1000	+.4	+.3	+2	+20
Lactating			+500	+20	+400	+400	+18	+2000	+.5	+.5	+5	+40

a. Source: U.S. Food and Drug Administration, *Nutritional Value of Foods*, Home and Garden Pamphlet 72. The U.S. RDA, formulated by the Food and Drug Administration, should not be confused with the RDA devised by the Food and Nutrition Board of the National Research Council. RDA levels are calculated to meet the nutritional needs of virtually all healthy people, but the U.S. RDA levels are slightly higher to approximate the greatest RDA needed. In most cases these figures are more than what is considered adequate for the maintenance of good nutrition. I chose to use the U.S. RDA here to demonstrate that these "higher than necessary" values are probably still much lower, with the exception of calcium, iron, and calories, than what most American women get in their diet.

b. These amounts of protein are recommended if you eat eggs, fish, meat, milk, and poultry. If you are a vegetarian and do not eat these foods, 65 grams of protein is recommended.

c. The increased requirements cannot be met by ordinary diets; therefore, the use of supplemental iron is recommended.

all that doesn't make you reconsider, think about this. Large doses of niacin (vitamin B_3) might actually block the release of free fatty acids and speed up the use of muscle sugar (glycogen) so that instead of burning fat when you run, you use up your sugar.

In addition to the side effects I've already discussed, vitamin B overdose can also result in peripheral neuropathies, including numbness, ataxia (uncoordinated muscle movements), and paralysis. Too much vitamin C, which is also water soluble, may cause kidney stones and gout. Instead of thinking that water-soluble vitamins are harmless, it's better to say that the toxicity caused by them is more easily alleviated by discontinuance than is the case with the fat-soluble vitamins.

Here's some more fuel for my fire. What about the impurities in vitamins? The FDA allows a 2 percent impurity level in synthesized vitamins as long as the impurities are nontoxic at the RDA level. But when these vitamins are taken in megadoses, the impurities may exceed the limits of safety.

"So," you ask, "is there *any* vitamin or mineral that an athlete might need more of?" Yes! Endurance exercise appears to have a depleting effect on iron, particularly if the individual is on a low-iron (vegetarian) diet or simply a low-calorie diet. Women of childbearing age and adolescent males are especially susceptible to iron deficiency. Does this mean the high-risk groups should take megadoses? Of course not. There are also bad effects from taking too much iron. However, a *modest* iron supplement is in order. Assume that your diet has some iron, in fact, almost enough. So taking a pill that supplies 25–50 percent of the RDA will be more than enough. I've never seen such a pill, so you may have to take one that supplies 100 percent. That will provide three or four times what you need, but it won't be in the toxic realm.

If you feel that your diet is not balanced, then one-a-day vitamins that meet RDA standards are probably a safe choice. To megadose on certain vitamins or minerals seems not only foolish

but extremely risky. Large doses can disrupt normal body functions or interfere with the action of other vitamins and minerals.
Some people say, "Who knows what good they may be doing?"
I say, "Do you know what bad they may be doing?" There's too
little evidence to support the possible benefits and too much data
confirming the harmful side effects to take the risk.

How to Gain Weight

I HOPE THE TITLE of this chapter caused you to do a double take. Are you thinking, "I don't need to *gain* weight. I'll just skip this chapter"? If you are, then hold on a minute! Maybe the fat on your body hides a skinny set of muscles. How would you look if most of your fat were removed? Is there a skinny, emaciated-looking body hiding under there? Many women are dissatisfied with their appearance even after fat loss because their muscles are either flabby or just too small.

All of us can picture a fat friend who lost weight through dieting alone. He or she looks slimmer but doesn't have the firmness of someone who lost fat with diet *and* exercise. This same softness is apparent when a thin person tries to *gain* weight by eating more. Skinny people should never try to fatten up, but they can fill out by adding muscle. If you build muscle, you usually gain some weight, and if you concentrate on *muscle* gain rather than *weight* gain you are more likely to be successful. *Muscle* gain enhances body contours, making men look stronger and improving women's curves. *Fat* gain hides all those beautiful lines under a layer of mush.

Whether you are naturally "too thin" because of anorexia or disease, or simply haven't used your muscles for many years, you should consider some muscle building. But if I had titled this chapter "How to Gain Muscle," many women would have skipped over it anyway. They think that muscle building is a man's thing. They conjure up images of sweaty bodies and grunting noises and decide it's not for them. But women need more muscle! Just as fat control isn't something that only fat people should practice, muscle building isn't something that only men, or only skinny people, should do.

Let's look at a sample woman:

> Total weight: 120 pounds
> Percentage of fat: 30
> Pounds of fat: 36
> Pounds of lean: 84

She has 84 pounds of lean, that is, fat-free tissue in her body. This lean is primarily bone and muscle, and the immediate question is, is 84 pounds a lot or a little for this woman? In the chart below you can see that 84 pounds of lean is approximately the midrange for women who are 5'3", but is low for women 5'7" and very low for women 5'10". If our sample woman were 5'3", she might look quite average. If she were 5'7", she would probably look slender or frail. A woman with only 84 pounds of lean at 5'7" would have small bones and/or small muscles.

Pounds of Lean Body Mass (Frame Size) for Women and Men

	5'0"	5'1"	5'2"	5'3"	5'4"	
Women	70–86	73–89	75–91	78–93	81–96	

	5'5"	5'6"	5'7"	5'8"	5'9"	5'10"
Women	83–99	86–102	90–105	93–109	95–115	98–119
Men	108–120	110–125	112–129	118–132	122–137	127–145

	5'11"	6'0"	6'1"	6'2"	6'3"
Men	133–153	137–163	140–168	143–176	145–183

The chart was compiled from my clinic records on the 20,000 people we have tested. It does not include anyone else's research, so it may have to be amended in time. In making the chart, we did not include those people with abnormally high or low body fat. It represents the range of lean in relatively fit people.

Approximately half of the people we test have more or less lean than shown on the chart for their height. Often you can see these differences just by looking at them. There are some great big men and women who you can tell have large bones and muscles and some thin people who have small bones and muscles. But some fool you; they look average, but the test shows that they have quite a lot or surprisingly little lean. It is hardest to guess the lean amounts of very fat people because their fat obscures their lean.

It used to be popular to categorize people by body type; a thin person was an ectomorph, a fat person was an endomorph, and someone with a large, muscular build was considered a mesomorph. These categories create problems. It's possible for one fat person to have very small bones and another to have very large bones. Is one an ectomorphic endomorph and the other a mesomorphic endomorph? To avoid all these tongue twisters, it makes more sense to simply classify a person as having a low, moderate, or high lean body mass.

Many people say to me, "I look normal, but you say my lean is large (or small). Is that good or bad?" In most cases, we feel the more lean the better. But there are exceptions. Take our sample woman again. If she is 5'9", her lean is below the range shown on the chart. But the immersion test doesn't distinguish between bone and muscle. If she was born with small bones, we can't expect her to add much muscle. On the other hand, if her bones are of average size but her muscle quantity or density is low, she can change dramatically. Large-boned people seem to add muscle easily.

There are distinct advantages to having lots of lean. We think you should strive to have a lean body mass (or frame) that is either within the range of the chart *or above it*. If you have a high

Bailey's Backpacking Formula

Summertime again, and he wants to go backpacking. You're not so eager. You remember last year. How your back ached. How tired you were! He told you to stop complaining. After all, he had read a magazine article that said women should carry about 20 percent less than men. And he was generous. He allowed you 25 percent less! This year you're saved. Ta-da! Enter the tried and tested Bailey Backpacking Formula! Here's what you do:

Get a body fat test for yourself and your partner. You'll need to find out your lean body weights and your fat weights. Here's my formula: carry a pack that is no heavier than one-half of your lean body weight. About now, you both are probably groaning. His lean weight is somewhere around 140 (a 70-pound backpack), and yours is around 90 (a 45-pound pack). But wait! You already carry a backpack all the time, day and night. That's right, your fat. Your fat weight should be included as part of the total backpack weight:

Backpack weight = ½ lean weight *minus* fat weight.

	Him	*You*
Total weight	170 lbs.	125 lbs.
% fat	18%	24%
Lean weight	140 lbs.	95 lbs.
Fat weight	30 lbs.	30 lbs.
Backpack weight	40 lbs.	18 lbs.

A woman, in general, should carry only about half as much weight as a man. Not only do men have much more muscle, but their lean-to-fat ratio is also considerably higher. (In the example above, both are toting the same "fat" backpack, but he has a lot more muscle with which to carry it.) Now you both may decide that the suggested pack weights are too light for what you need to have on the trip. Fine, carry more, but still try to have the man carry twice as much. At the end of the day you'll both be equally tired (or equally refreshed if you carried the recommended load!).

muscle mass, consider yourself lucky. You can consume more calories because it's muscle that burns up most of the calories you eat. More lean also means that you'll tend to be better at sports. Some women with a large lean mass aren't at all happy about it. To them, being healthy and strong is no asset if they are considered stocky, rugged, or big. They express a desire to be more "womanly." But today it's "in" to be a strong woman, as evidenced by the increase in the number of women body builders. Muscular women should be proud of their strength and enjoy the beauty of it. In any case, for both men and women, I think the amount of muscle you have (as reflected in your lean mass) is very important, and it is my prejudice to want you to increase it.

When I do body fat testing for a group, there's usually one man or woman in the group who is very thin. If it's a woman, her friends crowd around the immersion tank because they're certain her results will be about 10 percent fat. My staff and I smile to ourselves because we know she's more likely to be 19, 20, or even as high as 25 percent fat. If we are right, it's not that she has too much fat. Rather, she is thin because her lean is too low. Her friends say she is quite lean, but we say just the opposite: she doesn't have much lean at all. Her muscle mass is too low and she is, in fact, quite unlean. If I'm lucky, the same group will have a nicely muscled man or woman who sinks like a rock in the tank. A woman like this is usually 15 or 16 percent fat. These are the *lean* ones — their muscle mass is high.

If you've had a body fat test and you have less than thirty pounds of fat, that's good. But if your pounds of lean are on the low side for your height (according to the Lean Body Mass chart), I recommend muscle *building* through moderate to heavy weight lifting for people under age fifty and muscle *maintenance* through lighter weight lifting for people over fifty.

Some people, especially women, are concerned that weight lifting will make them too bulky. A few women have high levels of testosterone, which is responsible for bulky muscle. But this is rare. Most women need not fear this possibility. Their muscles will become more shapely rather than more bulky. The kind of bulk seen in female professional body builders requires hours and hours of effort. The average woman on a moderate body building program will not take on male characteristics.

Weight lifting is *not* a fat-burning exercise. Areas that are too thin or too flabby benefit from specific body building exercises that tone and tighten the underlying muscles. But if an area is just plain "too fat," don't rely on weight lifting to slim it down. Remember that fat is a localized symptom of a systemic disorder; it must be treated *systemically* with aerobic exercise to change muscle chemistry and with diet to reduce overall fat. There is no way you can eliminate fat selectively from one portion of your body. Fat is systemic and you lose it from *all* parts of your body. But you can *treat* localized areas of poor muscle development. Women can firm up flabby thighs or enhance the appearance of their bustline. Strengthening certain muscles will help you perform better in your favorite sport. I've seen pretty spectacular results from simple, selective muscle building.

Weight Lifting Advice for the Beginner

IN GENERAL, the rules for effective weight lifting haven't changed in a hundred years. The professionals argue about some subtleties, but the basics are the same. Weight lifting, unlike aerobic exercise, demands concentration. You have to think about the specific area and the specific muscles you are working. This requires a little of what I call "muscle sense," which women often lack. In the teenage years, when the girls are learning about mascara, the boys are busy flexing their muscles, and, from then on, it's more natural for the males to have muscle sense.

Here's a simple thing you can do to test your muscle sense. Lift one arm so that the elbow is slightly bent and the entire arm is parallel to the floor, as if you're getting ready to take a partner in the waltz. Now pretend you are pulling a giant beach ball toward your chest as hard as you can. With your other hand, feel the muscles in your chest above your breasts. Are they hard or soft? Now relax your arm. Can you flex those same muscles without lifting or tightening the arm muscles? If you can, you have muscle sense.

Concentrate on the muscle being worked and keep the action specific to that muscle. One of the excellent features of Nautilus-style weight lifting machines is that the design of each machine practically forces you to exercise only a specific muscle group. They help you to develop muscle sense. The equipment requires that your body be in such a position that you can't use the wrong muscles. The Nautilus curl machine is a great example of an isolated muscle exercise. When you see people doing curls with a barbell, they often "cheat," using their abdominal or back or shoulder muscles to lift the weight. On the Nautilus machine, however, it is almost impossible to use any muscle except the biceps.

Even if you don't want to be a member, get a friend to take you to a weight lifting place that specializes in machines. Go around their circuit just once, slowly and thoughtfully. Those circuits are designed to give every major muscle group the best possible workout in the least amount of time. I realize that women, especially those who are overweight, are reluctant to visit a weight lifting place. That's a shame, because the beginner who, on her own, is likely to bumble around for months, could acquire in a week at Nautilus a feeling of muscle sense: how much weight is correct, how hard to work, and how often to lift.

Isolating specific muscles is difficult for the beginner. At first, try working just three sets of muscles. For example, for a week just work on your biceps by doing curls with a three- or five-pound weight. Work your quadriceps (the upper thigh muscles) by doing twenty to thirty half squats. Isolate the abdominals by doing sit-ups in which you lift your upper body only a few inches off the floor, keeping the back flat and the knees bent. One of the surest ways to know whether you have succeeded in isolating a specific muscle group is a burning sensation in the area you are working. Additionally, you'll often have soreness in that area the following day. Biceps, quadriceps, and abdominals are easy to isolate, it's easy to create the "burn" in them, and next day soreness is readily apparent. As your muscle sense develops, you'll find you can learn to isolate and work the more difficult muscles such as the pectorals, triceps, and back.

Do not work a specific muscle group more often than every 48 hours. Your muscles need repair time after weight lifting. If you lift too often, you'll lose rather than gain muscle tissue.

Remember to breathe! This sounds silly, but beginners often hold their breath while lifting. This may raise your blood pressure, and you might even faint if you strain too hard. Get in the habit of inhaling deeply with the beginning of each movement and exhaling at its completion.

Heavy weights and few repetitions increase muscle mass. Light weights and more repetitions tone and firm muscle without increasing size. Let me stress again that it is rare for a woman to bulk up like a man, so don't be afraid of using weights that feel slightly heavy. When it comes to selecting the correct amount of weight for a specific exercise, the general rule is: pick a weight that you can lift ten times in a row. Suppose you are doing curls. Stand up straight, take a dumbbell in one hand (no! not your husband!), and curl your hand up toward your shoulder. If you can only do it once or twice, it's too heavy. If you can do it fifteen times nonstop, it's too light. Try different dumbbells until you get one that requires some effort for the tenth lift. The experienced weight lifter wants that tenth lift to be as difficult as possible. Not for you! Make that tenth lift hard but not herculean.

Each lift of the weight up to the shoulder and back down to straight arm is called a repetition, or "rep" if you are talking to a hotshot. Eight or ten repetitions nonstop is called a set. We recommend that you rest a few moments after a set, then do another, rest again, and do a final set. Obviously, the last lift of the last set is going to be the hardest. If you have done it right, tomorrow morning you will feel sore in that exact muscle, and you will be able to stare at it and flex it. You will never again wonder what I mean by muscle sense.

Always work the larger muscles first and the smaller ones later. If you exercise your biceps (relatively small muscles) first, they'll be too tired to assist with the chest workout later. A good general workout might follow this order: chest, shoulders, front thighs, back, back thighs, neck, biceps, triceps, calves.

I feel that supervision is mandatory for the novice weight lifter. This way you can avoid getting into bad habits, and you'll have someone to spur you on when you feel like giving up. Nautilus-type equipment is particularly good for the beginner because it encourages muscle isolation, and you are less likely to injure yourself. There are plenty of good books available on the subject, but hold off on using these until you have established a certain amount of muscle sense. Let your instructor design a program for you that works on all your muscles. Later, by referring to books, you can develop your own regime to emphasize or slim certain body parts.

Don't forget that you can do weight lifting without using weights. Sit-ups, push-ups, and leg lifts are all forms of weight lifting. Most good exercise classes include thirty to forty-five minutes of floor exercises that are like weight lifting. Just remember my number-one rule when you do them: isolate and concentrate on the muscle being worked. When you lie on your side to do leg lifts, for instance, be aware of which muscles you are working. Do you want the muscles on the front of the thigh to get the workout? If so, raise your leg to the front. Lifting your leg toward the back will work the buttock and hamstring muscles. If you want to work the muscles wrapping around the side of the leg, then you must raise your leg exactly parallel to the floor. In each instance the movement should be slow, while the muscle involved is flexed with maximum resistance to the direction of the movement. You can't just haphazardly fling your leg into the air and expect to get a shapely leg.

Muscle work, unlike aerobics, requires concentration. When you jog or do aerobic dancing, you can let your mind wander, and your body can be loose and free. But when you weight lift, your efforts must be controlled.

HOW TO TRACK
YOUR PROGRESS

How Fat or Fit Are You?

THE POINT SHOULD BE CLEAR by now that a weight loss program really means: FAT DECREASE coupled with FITNESS INCREASE. You need good ways to measure each of these.

It won't do to try to measure fat loss on your bathroom scale. When you buy a steak, do you select the lightest one you can find on the assumption that it must have the least fat? Sounds ridiculous, doesn't it? Yet that's what many people assume when they weigh themselves on the bathroom scale. If their weight is less, they think, then they must have lost some fat. But that lost weight may be water loss or muscle loss, and not fat.

Suppose two women decide to lose weight. The first woman goes on a radical diet and loses twenty pounds in a month. The second woman decides to exercise aerobically, diet sensibly, and do low-intensity weight lifting. At the end of the month the second woman has lost only eight pounds. The first woman seems to be more successful at losing weight. But who is more successful at losing *fat*? Body fat testing might show that the first woman has actually lost ten pounds of fat, seven pounds of water, and three pounds of muscle. The second woman also may have lost ten pounds of fat but *gained* two pounds of muscle. At the end of the month the first woman finds that it's harder than ever to keep her weight down because she has lost fat-burning muscle. The second woman can enjoy eating more food but won't gain weight because she has more muscle to burn up extra calories.

Body fat testing is almost essential to a proper weight control program. Measuring changes in your fitness level is equally important because the measurement is a monitor of all the metabolic changes you can expect. Fitness isn't simply how fast you can run or how much weight you can lift. Men often mistakenly equate fitness with these two abilities. If they can rip telephone books, then they must be fit. If they can run a hundred feet in ten seconds, then they must be fit. But too often they are *not* fit and end up having a heart attack.

Fitness encompasses a whole range of metabolic changes, in blood chemistry, the brain, the muscles, and cardiovascular condition, as well as in the body's ability to burn fat. To measure all these changes individually would require tedious and expensive laboratory procedures. But the chapter "The Best Possible Fitness Test" describes an indirect way of measuring them. If you are improving aerobically, then all the other changes are occurring too. I especially urge readers to take this fitness test and not scoff at its simplicity.

Get a body fat test. Measure your fitness. If you've read this far into the book yet neglect to do these two tests, you have wasted your time and money. These two measurements, done on a regular basis, give you all the information you need in order to evaluate the effectiveness of your fat control program.

Body Fat Testing Methods

FOR ABOUT TEN YEARS, I traveled throughout the United States and Canada with my portable water tank, testing all sorts of people: dentists, physicians, Weight Watchers, Mormons, marathoners. You name the group — I can probably tell you their average body fat. Today I seldom use the underwater immersion test. Enough people have been trained in this method that any medium-sized city can boast of at least one testing center. When I do include body fat analysis with my lectures, I now rely on measurements with skin calipers. They're not quite as accurate, but they allow me to test many more people with fairly reliable results.

If you are 20 percent fat, then obviously you are 80 percent lean. Body fat testing doesn't tell you where that 20 percent fat is located, although most women know pretty well where it is. The test also doesn't tell you what percentage of your lean is water or bone or muscle. When you lose or gain weight, the test can tell you what contributed to the change (loss or gain of fat or lean), but it can't tell you *where* the change occurred. Additionally, if you show a loss of lean, the test can't tell you if it is due to dehydration, muscle atrophy, bone mineral loss, or disease. Sophisticated laboratories now use CAT scans and neutron activation analysis, which can zero in on the position of fat depots. In addition, since they measure protein and calcium, they can estimate muscle and bone. But such tests are very expensive and are not currently available to the general public. The following methods are presently used:

Skin calipers. This method uses skin-fold measurements of subcutaneous fat to estimate total body fat. For average people the results are accurate within 3–4 percent; that is, a test reading of 15 percent means the individual is 11–19 percent fat. The underwater immersion is also reliable only within 3–4 percent. Thus for the average individual skin calipers can be considered an efficient tool. The major drawback of the method is that it measures subcutaneous fat only, unlike the water immersion test, which assesses *all* body fat. The test assumes that the amount of skin fat accurately reflects the amount of internal fat. Although this assumption is usually quite accurate, the operator should not rely on the results when testing either very fit athletes or thin, sedentary individuals. In the first type, the trained athlete, the calipers overestimate intramuscular fat and give body fat percentages 5–10 points higher than those obtained through water immersion. The opposite occurs with the nonathletic, "skinny" person. The calipers estimate a lower percentage of intramuscular fat than is obtained with water immersion.

Electrical impedance. This technique involves sending a small electrical current through the body and measuring the body's resistance to that current. Electricity travels easily through lean tissue but poorly through fat. Therefore, the more electrical resistance, the more fat a person has. As with skin calipers, the value of this method is that it does not require the person being tested to do anything. When impedance was first introduced, operators ran into many problems. Different machines produced different results, and even the same machine gave widely varying numbers on the same individual. By 1988 many of these problems had been ironed out, and results were reliable within 3–4 percent, the same as with skin calipers. However, I use and recommend calipers simply because they've been around longer and they're $5000 cheaper.

Ultrasound. This device sends a sound wave down through the skin and fat to the underlying lean dense tissues, where it bounces off and then returns to the machine. Essentially, the technique measures the thickness of skin and subcutaneous fat, just as the skin calipers do. The results are about the same as with the calipers, the accuracy is about the same, and the problems are the same. One big difference is that the ultrasound information is fed into a computer, which then produces a very elaborate printout with much more information than is justified by the input. The computer makes the test look more accurate than it really is.

Underwater immersion. For the general population, this is still considered the "gold standard" for body composition analysis. If the test is done correctly, the results will most closely reflect a person's actual fat and lean content. However, fear of water, retained air (in the lungs, intestines, or even the hair or clothing), or an unusual state of hydration will throw off the results. I once tested a man at 15 percent fat. During the following six months he exercised hard and was careful with his diet. He looked leaner, and my practiced eye estimated that he had dropped to 10 or 12 percent. However, he consumed three bowls of chili beans the night before the second test. He felt very bloated, and the intestinal gas that causes bloating made him float in the water tank. He tallied in at 23 percent. I was so sure his results were wrong that I tested him again a week later; minus the bloating, he was 12 percent.

Here's another way water tank results can be thrown off, even when run by an experienced operator. The bloated feeling that women experience before menstruation is not always fluid retention, as some people claim. Sometimes it is caused by gas in the intestines, resulting in a reading of 2–3 percent more body fat than is correct. Three days later, even if cramps are bad, the gas has disappeared and the percentage of fat is down to the woman's correct level.

People who have done the dunk tank sometimes try to manipulate the results the second time. This is fun for my staff because people usually do the wrong things and make their results worse. For example, some don't eat for two days before the test. They may lose several pounds and assume the test will show less body fat. However, their weight loss is mostly water, which comes from the lean part of the body. If their lean mass is artificially depressed by dehydration, then their fat mass is a higher percentage of total weight and the percentage of fat goes up.

To get worse results on your water immersion test, do the following:
1. Don't drink water. Get dehydrated.
2. Eat beans and other gas-producing foods or beverages prior to testing.
3. Exercise to exhaustion prior to the test.
4. Don't blow out all your air when underwater.

To get better results, do the following:
1. Eat a low-fat diet for six months prior to the test.
2. Do aerobic exercise for six months prior to the test.
3. If you need more lean, add weight lifting to your exercise program.
4. Eat and drink normally prior to the test, but don't stuff yourself.
5. Sew little lead weights inside your swimsuit.

Race, age, sex. During the years of my "floating road show," I tested more than 25,000 people. Even though I admonish my audiences not to judge body fat from appearance, I got pretty good at estimating the percentage of fat from visual and tactile data. The novice eye is fooled by a person's size; if she's thin, she must be low in fat, and if she's large, she must be high. The "pinch an inch" test was popular for a while. If you could gather up more than an inch of flesh around your midsection, then it was time to switch to the diet drinks. I don't bother with these superficial measurements. I get a good grip on the waist or the upper arm and feel for deep-down muscular solidity. I can usually predict a person's body fat to within 1–2 percent of the water tank result.

So I was perturbed when I kept missing the mark with black people. A black man would come in who looked and felt a little fat. I would predict his body fat at 18 percent, but the tank would show he was 14 percent. With black men and women, my visual assessment was always too high by 3–4 percent. It turns out that blacks have denser bones and muscles than whites, so they are heavier in water. Instead of striving for 22 percent fat, the ideal for white women, black women should be 19 percent. In 1985 new formulas were derived for blacks based on their greater lean density.

Orientals have lighter bones than whites, so my mistakes were just the opposite. Their lower lean density makes it easier for them to float. If the standard Caucasian formula is used, then Orientals should be allowed a 3 percent increase in fat percentage.

And here's an observation that I haven't seen verified in technical journals, but I assure you it will be proven one of these days: freckled redheads, just like blacks, have greater lean densities. They, too, need to aim for 3 percent less fat if the standard Caucasian formula is used. Have you noticed how blacks and the redheaded Irish gravitate to contact sports such as football and boxing? They're so solid it's hard to make a dent in them. The lighter-framed Orientals, on the other hand, excel in sports that aren't weight-dependent, such as swimming and gymnastics.

Ideal Body Fat Percentages
(using standard Caucasian formulas)

	Men	Women
White	15	22
Black	12	19
Oriental	18	25
Redhead	12	19

The original percentages were derived from cadaver studies of young white males. Until there are standards that take into account racial differences, it makes sense to modify the results obtained when using the Caucasian calculation.

Assessment of children also poses problems. Children have more water and less bone mineral in their lean body mass than adults. Thus the standard formula may overestimate the real amount of body fat by 4–5 percent. Most young children average 15 percent fat. With the onset of puberty, males show dramatic increases in lean while females slowly add fat. By the time they graduate from high school, healthy, athletic boys are 10–12 percent and the girls are 19–22 percent.

Similarly, the loss of bone mineral and muscle in adults over fifty makes the standard formula less reliable for this group. A high body fat percentage may be indicative of low lean rather than high fat.

Look again at the chart "Women's Body Fat Percentages" in the chapter "Healthy Women *Do* Jiggle." Notice that 19–25 percent fat is *healthy* and that 30–33 percent fat is *average*. Ten or more years ago, when body fat testing was new, the assumption was often made that very low body fat — near 6 percent — was ideal for athletes, both male and female. Some coaches designed diets to produce 6 percent fat in their athletes and even fined or dismissed players who didn't achieve it. In most instances, 6 percent fat is just enough to maintain health in men and much too low for women. There are exceptions, but most male athletes range from 5 to 13 percent, and most female athletes are between 12 and 22 percent. If professionals in the field make these mistakes, it shouldn't be surprising that untrained individuals do the same.

Nonetheless, I am dismayed by the number of people who misinterpret their body fat test results. They mistake the *ideal* fat percentages for *average* fat percentages. They are unhappy with what they think are only mediocre results, when in reality they are at optimum health and fitness.

> Gradual weight loss is the safest way to ensure fat reduction without muscle loss. I recommend no more than ½ percent fat loss per month.

I also worry that people take their results too literally. If a woman is 26 percent fat and we tell her she needs to lose seven pounds to be 22 percent, that number becomes a dictum. She may go to extremes of exercise and diet and lose seven pounds of muscle rather than fat. She may be quite lean and actually need to build muscle rather than lose fat. And it's possible that the number we give her is not exactly correct. As we have seen in the above examples, the color of her skin, her age, the time of the month, or even the color of her hair could affect the results.

If you have had a body fat test, please do not consider the number you got to be an absolute. Remember, the percentage could be off by 3–4 percent. If your percentage of fat is too high, aim for a *gradual* downward change. I recommend losing no more than one-half of one percent fat per month. If your diet and exercise habits are good but you repeatedly test 2–3 percent over the ideal, don't worry about it! You may be one of those people who don't quite fit the formula. Instead of beating yourself physically and emotionally, accept the number you got as *your* set point and endeavor to maintain that percentage over the years.

The Best Possible Fitness Test

A CAR GOING SIXTY miles an hour is traveling one mile a minute. That is a one-minute mile. Roger Bannister was the first person to break the four-minute mile. When I was a graduate student at MIT, I barely managed to run a six-minute mile. I don't know how fast I could run a mile right now, and since I'm in my mid-fifties, I don't intend to find out. But I do know that the pace of my usual daily jog ranges from an eight-minute mile when I feel great to a ten-minute mile when I'm at a higher altitude or I'm feeling really down. Women who are overweight may take fifteen minutes to cover a mile. And some need a half-hour to go the same distance.

In twenty minutes, a very fit few can comfortably run four miles. Someone who is very unfit may be able to cover only one mile in twenty minutes and still be comfortable. The point is that people who walk, jog, or run fairly routinely have established an exercise pace. They have a pace that feels comfortable, that doesn't leave them feeling exhausted or cause soreness the next day.

It's important to distinguish between this comfortable pace and the pace you might be able to attain if you really pushed, by being in a race, for example. Your daily exercise pace should be the *fastest* pace you can maintain for an extended period — say a half-hour — without feeling exhausted or sore. Sometimes in my lectures I really shake up the cardiologists present by pausing between the first and second half of the next sentence. "The first day you even begin a walking/jogging program, you should go as fast as you can go . . . *without* exceeding the pace that you could sustain comfortably for a half-hour, *without* going so fast as to cause soreness tomorrow." The cardiologists almost have a stroke worrying about all the unfit people in the room running madly into a heart attack — until they hear the second part of the sentence.

If you follow the rules of the whole sentence, you *won't* suffer anything, you *will* be doing a good thing for your body, and by definition, you will have done an *aerobic* exercise. A bad mistake made by many beginning joggers is that they run as fast as they can for one or two minutes, then walk for a few minutes to get their breath back before going into another one- or two-minute sprint. *They're* the ones who fill the cardiologists' offices. It is much safer for the novice to maintain a steady, slow pace — one she can *comfortably* handle for fifteen to thirty minutes without needing to rest.

Now, here's how to do my "best possible fitness test." Everyone, I repeat, *everyone,* even if walking or jogging is not your thing, should do a walk/jog exercise for several days in order to establish your *fastest comfortable* pace and your heart rate at that pace. Each day, after you have been walking or jogging for about fifteen minutes, stop and take your pulse for 6 seconds, as described in *Fit or Fat?* Multiply by 10 to get heart rate in beats per minute. Don't worry if the heart rate you get is much lower or higher than you expected it to be. (Refer to the chapter "Heart Rate As an Indicator of Exercise"). If you have been exercising at your *fastest comfortable* pace, then you have determined your correct aerobic heart rate better than could be done in most laboratories.

One of the women in my center had trouble with this concept at first. She is forty years old, and the heart rate charts say that

144 is her correct aerobic pulse. When she jogs, however, she is quite comfortable at a pulse of 165. Aerobic instructors are forever telling her to slow down, but when she does, she doesn't "get any exercise." Well, she has a small heart that goes very fast for her age, so she can sustain 165 beats per minute for a half-hour without discomfort. Since you, my reader, may also have a smaller (or larger) than average heart, you must also establish your own personal aerobic heart rate.

I want every reader to establish her aerobic pulse rate. Check it for three or four days in a row. Then figure out your minutes per mile while maintaining your aerobic pulse.

This is the easiest, cheapest, most accurate, and practical fitness test ever invented. We have every woman at our center do the test approximately once a month. Inevitably, their minutes per mile drop; that is, while walking or running at the exact same heart rate of a month ago, they cover a mile in fewer minutes. A fatter person might drop from a fifteen-minute mile to a fourteen-minute mile while maintaining the same heart rate. Our joggers may improve from a ten-minute mile to a nine-and-a-half-minute mile while continuing an aerobic pace.

There's a subtle but extremely significant difference between my fitness test and most others. Most fitness books have fancy charts based on age and sex. You can look up your appropriate category and the charts will tell you, for example, that you're very fit if you can run a mile in six minutes, moderately fit if you do it in nine, and very unfit if it takes you fifteen minutes. The fallacy of these charts is that they are measuring *an*aerobic ability, not aerobic ability. You are encouraged to run the fastest you can (*not* your *fastest comfortable* pace) in order to get a better rating. Such a test is not a true measure of your fitness, and it's dangerous. Simply from determination, will power, and strength one person may run faster than her friend who is just as aerobically fit.

My test is a true measure of aerobic fitness. You *must* perform the test at a comfortable pace, or it will not be accurate. I don't give you numbers or charts to measure yourself against, because I don't want you to compare yourself with others. You should compare yourself only with you. If you can jog a mile this year faster than you did last year, your fitness has improved. Or if you can jog a mile in ten minutes when you are thirty-five years old and can still do it in ten minutes when you are forty, then your fitness has improved.

When women first come to our center, they want to lose weight and don't care about their fitness. They don't care how long it takes them to walk a mile. We manage to convince them — we practically brainwash them — to accept our fitness approach. We get them to realize that their metabolism, or set point, or body chemistry, is changing so that they won't gain weight again. Please put yourself through this fitness test from time to time, knowing that as your aerobic minutes per mile improves, you are becoming a fat-burning animal.

OTHER ASPECTS
OF PHYSIOLOGY

Stress and Endorphins

THERE ARE TABLES that list the most stressful life changes. The higher an event is on the scale, the more stressful it is supposed to be. If two or more of the events happen at the same time, the stress is compounded. I recently had six of the events occur within a four-month period! My body reacted with one cold after another, and I had frequent bouts of depression.

Sometimes people feel "stressed out," yet they can't point to a specific major upset as the cause. They can't figure out why they're anxious, tense, irritable, or fatigued. It may turn out that a seemingly small daily stress rather than a major life stress is the cause. When something really bad happens to you, friends and family usually gather to lend support. You have an outlet for your feelings; you're *supposed* to be unhappy. But the day-by-day stresses — the ones that aren't supposed to bother you — can take a real toll.

It's the small chronic stresses that are the hardest to evaluate. A physician may easily overlook the real cause of an individual's emotional stress if he looks only at a chart of large stresses. Personally, I believe one of the most discomforting stressful conditions occurs when no one else understands the stress that you feel. In fact, your friends may make fun of you for feeling stress about something they find pleasant. For example, your husband may be friendly and full of good will toward everyone, and he expects

Stress Inducers

Major life changes	*Chronic "little stresses"*
Death or loss of a loved one	Family conflict
Serious illness or accident	I hate my job
Divorce or separation	Lack of time
Death of a close relative	Too much responsibility
Getting fired or laid off work	No one understands why I am stressed
Marriage	Sexual difficulties
Major personal property loss (fire, theft, vandalism)	Rush-hour traffic
New household member	

you to be the same way. You feel that you have to be "up" all the time just to please him. At parties, he is energized by all the people while you feel drained. All your friends comment on how lucky you are to be married to such a man. You smile and agree, yet deep down, you feel very uncomfortable and can't understand why.

What is stressful to some people may be enjoyable to others. For me, travel on any kind of public transportation is stressful. I hate airplanes, buses, taxis, whatever. Adjusting my schedule to someone else's timetable upsets me. In contrast, driving calms me down immediately. Lea, my co-author, is just the opposite. She avoids driving whenever possible, preferring what I call the "interminable terminal wait." Reading a book while waiting for an airplane relaxes her but drives me crazy.

Recognizing what is stressful *to you* is very helpful. Even if you can't change the source of the stress, you can change the way you feel about it. I have a dental hygienist friend who felt that it was *her* fault if a patient returned with bleeding gums. If she taught that patient how to floss his teeth so that the bleeding would stop, then she felt she was a failure if, after six months, he hadn't stuck with the program. She had to learn that some people won't change their habits no matter how good the change may be for them. She needed to count *her* successes rather than dwell on *their* failures. I suggested that she keep a record of how many people had improved over the last six months. When she did this, she was surprised that 80 percent had healthier mouths. She had been putting a lot of negative energy into her work when she could have been congratulating herself for a job well done.

These hidden, day-by-day issues can lead to very real physical ailments, including headaches, backaches, irritable bowel, and stomach ulcers. Changes in the blood vessel walls in response to constant stressful stimuli may result in high blood pressure. Even depression, premenstrual syndrome, anorexia, and bulimia have been linked, in various ways, to stress.

One of the best ways to reduce the symptoms of stress is with exercise. When laboratory rats are repeatedly faced with stressful situations, their heart rates increase and they develop high blood pressure. Researchers have found that when these rats are put on a running wheel, their stress is lowered; their heart rate is reduced, and their blood pressure drops. People with borderline hypertension have been able to lower blood pressure with aerobic exercise. Although the causes of stress may be mental, these are *physical* problems that are curbed with *physical* activity. It's as if exercise treats the physical problem itself.

As a bonus, exercise also seems to have an effect on your emotional reaction to stress. It does this by altering your mood. Fit people are usually in high spirits after a lengthy exercise, sometimes to the point of elation or joy. This feeling is associated with the presence of endorphins, which are released by the pituitary gland in the brain. The word "endorphin" is a combination of "endo" and "morphine," meaning endogenously produced morphine. Endorphins are the body's natural pain reliever. It may be that the brain interprets exercise as a form of "pain." Or it may be that the rise in fatty acids caused by long, gentle exercise acidifies the blood, which triggers the release of endorphins. In any case, one gets from exercise a natural high similar to a drug high but with none of the bad side effects. People who do long, continuous, gentle exercise enjoy the most effective stress therapy known to man.

How long and how hard do you have to exercise to get the endorphin high? Most researchers have found that moderate-intensity exercise lasting at least twenty to thirty minutes produces the greatest increase of blood endorphins. In stationary bicycle studies, subjects pedaled for eight minutes at 25 percent of their maximum exercise capacity followed by eight minutes at 50 percent, and then by eight minutes at 75 percent. The level of endorphins in the blood did not change during the 25 percent and 50 percent bouts. But it rose significantly during the 75 percent period. Then, ironically, if the subjects continued to exercise to exhaustion, the endorphin level dropped dramatically. It's as if the body were saying, "If you're going to exercise *this* hard, you must be in trouble. Maybe a bear is chasing you. Whatever it is, this is no time to be high!" This seems to provide yet another reason to exercise slowly, aerobically. During high-stress situations — running *too* fast — your body can't afford to have your brain tripping off into fantasyland.

You may have wondered whether the release of endorphins in the study above was triggered by the intensity of exercise (75 percent) or simply by the time elapsed (the cyclists had exercised about twenty minutes). Most researchers feel that it's a combination of the two. Twenty to thirty minutes of exercise at 60–80 percent maximum seems to produce the best results, but longer duration and lower intensity will also work. The only thing that doesn't work is short, high-intensity workouts.

So there you have it. Exercise can lessen physical reactions to stress. And in a way it also eliminates the stress itself. No, it doesn't change your husband or your job or your children. It won't make them go away. It *does* change your perception of situations so that they no longer seem so stressful.

Depression

DEPRESSION CAN BE either *reactive* or *endogenous*. All of us, at one time or another, have felt depressed because of some life change. Loss of a job, death of a close relative, even prolonged illness can cause temporary despondency. This is *reactive* depression, a normal reaction to a particular stressful event.

Women suffer from endogenous depression nearly four times as much as men. No one knows why. One of the reasons could be a yielding to social expectations; it's okay for a man to react angrily to a stressful situation, but a woman is "expected" to be ladylike and suppress hostile feelings. If a woman has to constantly reprogram her natural feelings and reactions into unnatural, but socially acceptable, behavior, depression certainly could result. Heredity also plays a strong role. If you have or have had bouts of depression, there is a 40–50 percent chance that another close family member — parent, brother, sister, grandparent — has also had problems with depression. Often it is the women in the family tree who have the disorder. Is there a genetic factor that favors female depression?

Many researchers believe that although heredity and social pressure may be associated with depression, its true cause is biological. The female hypothalamus may be more sensitive to alterations in certain chemicals produced by nerve cells. Most likely, depression results from a combination of these three factors. Whatever the reason, many, many women are depressed!

Endogenous depression is believed to originate from a biochemical abnormality in the brain. Unlike reactive depression, there is no apparent reason for it. The sufferer frequently feels guilty about being depressed because "there's nothing really wrong." Endogenous depression often affects one's sleep habits; the individual either can sleep only a couple of hours a night, or she sleeps ten to twelve hours a day. The sex drive may be lost. Appetite is affected, and overeating or undereating is common. One of the classic signs of endogenous depression is its cyclic nature; it seems to peak at the same time every day. If a person has reactive depression, the mood stays more or less the same throughout the day, sometimes worse, sometimes better, depending on outside stimuli. But with endogenous depression there is a definite pattern. Some people wake up happy and gradually get more and more depressed as the day wears on. With others, it's the opposite. They feel better and better throughout the day and dread going to sleep at night, knowing they'll wake up miserable. Endogenous depression may last a few months or may go on for years. It may vanish spontaneously and then, just as mysteriously, reappear.

To someone who has known only reactive depression, it is hard to understand a sufferer of endogenous depression. "Why doesn't she just snap out of it?" is the common suggestion. Or, "If she would just exercise or read or make new friends, she wouldn't feel so depressed." Why doesn't she have the ability to control it? Most people with endogenous depression *have* tried to rid themselves of it. Exercise sometimes gives temporary alleviation, as do self-help books or group therapy. But the depression always seems to be there. As one person put it, "I have two moods: depressed and blank. If I'm not feeling down, I'm not feeling anything at all."

The two brain chemicals usually associated with endogenous depression are norepinephrine and serotonin. Researchers aren't sure whether the body doesn't know how to properly utilize these neurotransmitters or whether not enough are being manufactured. Whatever the reason, an imbalance of these two chemicals seems to be responsible for all the symptoms of endogenous depression. In the last few years physicians have had remarkable success in treating this form of depression with antidepressants, which seems to substantiate the theory that it is chemically rather than psychologically based. Antidepressants don't seem to help those with reactive depression, but they dramatically affect those with endogenous depression. More than 80 percent of the time symptoms disappear or are greatly reduced.

The lay public has a lot of misconceptions about antidepressants. Many think they are a sort of "happy pill" or a tranquilizer. Not so. They do not cover up feelings or induce artificial moods. They correct an underlying chemical imbalance so that the person feels normal again. Apathy disappears, making the individual able to cope with events that previously caused overwhelming feelings of hopelessness. If a normal person takes an antidepressant, she feels no changes at all other than the usual side effects of dry mouth and possible constipation. It doesn't alter one's mood the way marijuana or cocaine does. But for a person with endogenous depression, it's a wonderful drug. In other words, if the chemicals in the brain are normal, the user is unaffected by the antidepressant. If the chemicals are imbalanced, the drug puts things back in proper working order.

If endogenous depression has genetic and/or biochemical origins, is there much sense in pushing exercise as part of the treatment? Yes! The position taken by most physicians today is that any effective treatment program should include exercise. Reactive depression certainly responds to exercise. But exercise also affects moderate — not severe — endogenous depression. Many psychiatrists report that running three times a week is just as effective as traditional psychotherapy in the handling of mild to moderate depression. Exercise is the most reliable mood elevator known to man. Exercise stimulates the production of endorphins, which heighten mood and relieve pain. Moreover, the level of norepinephrine increases during exercise, with a surge of the chemical right afterward. When you exercise, your body makes its own drugs, and you can practice self-induced pharmacological treatment.

The mental changes that come from exercise are not solely the result of chemical fluctuations in the brain. Your mental attitude also changes as you become more confident of your abilities. Any time you set goals and achieve them through regular practice and discipline, you have feelings of mastery. You have replaced negative habits with positive ones. You have power. Women often feel frustrated in their efforts to gain equality in their work environment or their home life. Through exercise, women can get an inner sense of equality that no one can take away. *You* have control. *You* have self-worth.

When you're feeling depressed, it's awfully hard to think about exercising. If you've been exercising all along, you have the discipline to get out and run or swim or bicycle even though you really don't want to. You're saddened by some event but you know that exercise can help you get through it. But if you're depressed and you haven't made a commitment to exercise, it's not easy to propel yourself into action. Ask a friend to help you overcome your inertia and apathy. If you know that your mood gets worse at a certain time of day, arrange to exercise with your friend about an hour before that time. Be careful about whom you select for this. You don't want a competitive type; you need someone who encourages but doesn't push.

One reason for depression is setting unrealistic goals that you can't achieve. Don't do the same with your exercise by setting uncompromising standards. Instead, enjoy it! Be a runner, not a racer. Notice how good the sun feels on your face. If you're pushing yourself too much and breathing too hard, slow down! You shouldn't be thinking about how hard it is to get air in and out of your lungs but rather how refreshing that air feels on your skin or how good it smells. As with the physiological changes I'll be discussing later, psychological changes occur with *time* rather than intensity. You're better off jogging or walking for a comfortable thirty to forty-five minutes than running hard for fifteen minutes. In fact, it's been shown that overtraining or high-intensity training sometimes leads to depression! Some people become overdependent on the good feelings they get and become exercise abusers. They exercise through pain, injury, and sickness, getting more and more fatigued. Neglecting family and job in a futile search for that elusive high, they end up in a permanently bad mood.

A popular expression says, "Exercise is medicine." How true! The strength of fitness lies in its ability to prevent. But like some new miracle drug, it also treats symptoms. Imagine the lucky scientist who discovers a drug that prevents cancer. If that drug also relieved the symptoms of cancer for those who already had it, the scientist would surely win the Nobel Prize. Exercise is like that. It not only prevents but also treats.

Anorexia and Bulimia

KATHY WAS A MYSTERY to me. A very attractive woman and not overweight, she attended one of the six-week courses that I give several times a year. But she was overly intense about the course material. She took lots of notes, always came to class early and stayed late, and asked penetrating questions. Her questions were all food oriented, although she already knew much more about food than my average student. Finally one evening after class, I bugged her a little about her preoccupation with food, and her story came out. She spoke hesitantly at first, then more quickly, and finally, out of this pretty girl came a torrent of misery.

"For over seven years," she said, "I've been bulimic. It started very suddenly when I was in college. I had been depressed for a few weeks, and one afternoon I had an overwhelming urge to eat ice cream. I bought a half gallon, intending to eat a dishful, but I couldn't stop until I had eaten the whole container! I felt pretty nauseated and ashamed of myself, but I figured my body must have needed it since I hadn't been eating much. But the next day it happened again. And the next day, and the next. I couldn't control it. About four in the afternoon I just had to gorge on something sweet and fattening. I wasn't even hungry! It was just an uncontrollable urge to stuff something, anything, in my mouth. I must have been eating over 5000 calories a day!

"Within two weeks I gained twenty pounds. Even though I hated the way I was getting fat, I couldn't stop the binging. So I tried laxatives. At first they worked great. I'd sneak out like a thief in the night and buy a cartload of goodies, gobble them all up in a matter of hours, then finish off with a few laxatives and be rid of everything by morning. After a few weeks of this, the laxatives began to lose their effect. In spite of taking up to fifty a day, I started to gain weight again.

"That's when I tried vomiting. At first it was hard. But then I guess your body gets trained, and all I had to do was think about vomiting and I would. I was throwing up about fifteen times a day! My weight plummeted. My friends and family got really worried at one point because I dropped to ninety-five pounds. So I learned to let some of the food stay with me — I guess you'd call it selective purging.

"This kept on for about six years. And all that time no one knew there was anything wrong. It was like a shameful secret — I'd lock myself in my apartment and eat like a pig. Sure, there would be periods when everything would be normal, sometimes as long as two months, but then, back it would come like something out of a horror movie. And it *was* horrible! All I thought about was food. I didn't have any dates. I was afraid that if we went out to dinner, I'd turn into some maniacal bloated creature, gobbling my food and then devouring my date's. Besides, I wasn't interested in men, anyway, just food.

"I can remember a period of several weeks when each day I consumed a gallon of ice cream, six chocolate eclairs, and one or two bags of cookies. I got so ashamed and disgusted with myself, I just wanted to give up. I remember sitting on my kitchen floor, crying, surrounded by empty ice cream cartons and cookie wrappers and trying to decide the easiest way to kill myself.

"One day my best friend happened to show up and caught me in the middle of all the evidence, crying to myself. Thank God, she managed to pry the story out of me. She made me really mad because she told my family and some other close friends. But all together, they managed to convince me to get professional help and got me into a hospital that specializes in eating disorders. I was put on a ward with twelve other women who were either bulimic or anorexic. What a wacky group! One of the goals of the nurses was to get us to eat three meals a day. The anorexics would practically be forced to eat while the bulimics would gladly have devoured everything. Then we'd all be watched constantly to be sure we kept those meals down. Some girls learned to throw up in the shower while others would try to get rid of the calories by exercising to exhaustion.

"They put me on antidepressants and that really seemed to help. In two or three weeks I felt much better about myself so that I could be treated as an outpatient. Finally, I felt enough in control to be released completely. Without the constant dread of my daily binge I can enjoy life again. It's like being a little kid all over. Everything seems so new. It's been about nine months now since my last binge, the longest I've ever lasted, so I'm feeling pretty confident that I've got it licked.

"I've been taking your Fit or Fat classes to learn how to eat and exercise right. My body has been through so much trauma the last few years, it needs all the help I can give it."

Kathy's story seems incredible unless you have heard it, as I have, from dozens of women, or even hundreds. How can a woman eat that much food when she is not even hungry? The stories from anorexic women are equally bizarre. These emaciated women will not eat even though they are starving. Bulimia and anorexia have been lumped together in the press so often that many people don't know the difference. And, indeed, there are many similarities. In fact, about one in four anorexics engages in bulimic behavior. Both diseases are thought to have biological origins that are triggered by environmental stimuli. Both seem to have a hereditary link to other psychiatric disorders. Both occur predominantly in women. Bulimic women and anorexic women often use the same methods — vomiting, purging, excessive ex-

What Are Anorexia Nervosa and Bulimia?[a]

The patient with anorexia nervosa:

A. Has an intense fear of becoming fat. This fear of fat does not decrease even when she has lost significant amounts of weight.

B. Continues to "feel fat" even though emaciated.

C. Refuses to maintain a normal body weight for her age and height.

D. Has no known physical illness that could account for the weight loss.

The patient with bulimia:

A. Has recurrent episodes of binge eating (rapid consumption of a large amount of food in a discrete period of time, usually less than two hours).

B. Engages in at least three of the following:

1. Consumes high-calorie, easily ingested food during a binge.

2. Eats inconspicuously during a binge.

3. Terminates eating episodes through abdominal pain, sleep, social interruption, or self-induced vomiting.

4. Repeatedly attempts to lose weight with severely restrictive diets, self-induced vomiting, or use of cathartics or diuretics.

5. Shows frequent weight fluctuations of more than ten pounds because of alternating binges and fasts.

C. Is aware that the eating pattern is abnormal and is afraid of being unable to stop eating voluntarily.

D. Feels depressed and has self-deprecating thoughts following eating binges.

E. Does not have anorexia nervosa or any known physical disorder.

a. Adapted from American Psychiatric Association, *Diagnostic and Statistical Manual of Mental Disorders*, 3rd ed. (Washington, D.C.: American Psychiatric Association, 1980).

ercise — to rid their bodies of fat. And either bulimia or anorexia can result in sudden death from a heart attack caused by an electrolyte imbalance.

It is estimated that about 3 percent of the female population suffers from binge eating, as compared with the 1 percent that has or has had anorexia. Bulimics don't get the same media attention because, like Kathy, they learn to regulate their weight within "acceptable" limits so that they can hide their problem for years. There are lots of undiagnosed bulimics out there who carry on useful lives and act quite normal. As a result, you have probably heard less about bulimia, even though it is much more prevalent. Friends may be unaware of the problem, but the bulimic herself knows quite well that she isn't normal.

Anorexics, on the other hand, don't believe anything is wrong with them. How can a woman starve to the point of looking like a skeleton, be terrified of food, yet think nothing is wrong with herself?

Why are both disorders more common in women? There are lots of guesses. Some people blame it all on social or environmental factors. Women feel constantly pressured to be thinner, they deal with food more than men, and they are more likely to diet and binge than men. Psychological factors may make body image seem more important to a woman than to a man. A few researchers believe the cause is biological, that anorexia and bulimia are symptoms of a larger, underlying psychiatric disorder. Bulimia, in particular, seems to be definitely linked to chronic depression, another problem that is far more common in women than men. Researchers are finding that bulimics respond quite well to antidepressants. Within three weeks, the daily cyclic urge to binge usually disappears. Unfortunately, as of this writing, no drug has been found to be useful in the treatment of anorexics. It may be a psychological rather than a chemical disorder.

Bulimics and anorexics are truly not tuned in to their bodies. But the loose connection is beyond their control and requires medical help. Too often, well-meaning friends try to help them with friendly but ineffective counseling. It would be ludicrous to tell them to binge from the Target Diet or to exercise more, when they are probably putting in three hours of running a day. Diagnosed anorexia and bulimia *must* be treated by a professional.

I'm particularly alarmed by women who aren't true anorexics or bulimics but who "play" with these ideas. These are the ones who think it's fashionable to eat all they want and then throw it up. Or they diet constantly even though they aren't fat in the first place. Not only are they taking the risk of triggering the anorexic/bulimic mechanism, but they're being just plain stupid. Teenage girls are the most likely to do this and are the most likely to become truly anorexic or bulimic. Constant peer pressure, parental pressure, and advertising pressure really push young girls into potentially dangerous diet techniques. Anorexia and bulimia are common enough without asking for trouble.

PMS

PREMENSTRUAL SYNDROME (PMS) is one of the oldest and most common afflictions known to women and, secondarily, to men. "When my wife has PMS, she's not the only one who suffers!" For most women, symptoms are usually mild — fatigue, irritability, anxiety, bloating. But for some, PMS is not mild, it's debilitating, causing severe depression, panic attacks, and even violent behavior. If 90 percent of women *worldwide* experience PMS symptoms to some degree, one begins to wonder whether it is an abnormal condition at all. Maybe it's a normal phenomenon, as "normal" as menstrual cramps. Menstrual cramps are associated with a positive body function, the shedding of the endometrial lining. Perhaps PMS is also related to some body change, and women are "supposed" to have it.

Some women believe that their PMS is due to a vitamin deficiency or to hypoglycemia. It's popular to say, "I have a hormone imbalance" or "I'm retaining fluids." Men sometimes feel that women are just too emotional. None of these theories have been verified by scientific research. In 1988 the National Institutes of Health (NIH) did a comprehensive study of PMS in several hundred women and disproved all of these ideas. It was shown that the hormone levels of women with PMS are *no different* from those who do not have PMS. Women who retain water do not have stronger symptoms. And psychological profiles show no difference between those who suffer from PMS and those who don't.

No definite cause has been shown for PMS. However, research suggests that neurointermediate lobe peptides may be involved. In practical terms, that term means endorphins. As I explained earlier, endorphins act on the body in much the same way as morphine. Whenever the body is experiencing pain, the level of endorphins in the blood rises. They not only relieve pain but, at the same time, give pleasurable sensations. Doctors can attest to the amazing effects of these self-produced pain relievers.

Endorphins are also released during extended periods of exercise (see the chapter "Stress and Endorphins") and are responsible for the "runner's high" you've heard about. People with anorexia have higher levels of endorphins, which may be one reason treatment is so difficult. The anorexic derives physical pleasure from the pain of starvation. The pleasure outweighs the pain, and she becomes very resistant to any measures taken to thwart these sensations.

But how can endorphins be related to PMS? The symptoms women experience before menstruation are certainly not pleasurable! Here is the connection. Many women, though not most, experience a sharp abdominal pain at ovulation. It is now thought that hundreds, or thousands of years ago, all women felt this pain at ovulation, which triggered a strong release of endorphins. Over time the ovulation pain has gradually diminished, but the body's conditioned response to it has not. Endorphins continue to be released when ovulation occurs. Like morphine, endorphins are addicting. Runners who can't run for a few days miss their "fix" and experience the withdrawal symptoms of irritability and depression. Similarly, all the various PMS symptoms may actually be signs of withdrawal from the sudden, brief midcycle surge of endorphins. With the pain of menstruation, more endorphins are released and the symptoms disappear.

According to this theory, the menstrual cycle is as follows:

1. First two weeks: no PMS
2. Ovulation: endorphin release

3. Last two weeks: endorphins diminish, PMS intensifies as the menstrual period approaches
4. Menstrual cramps: pain releases more endorphins, PMS disappears

The endorphin explanation of PMS is still only a theory, and even if it is proven correct, it still leaves the question of what practical things a woman can do about PMS. Advice in the past has been less than helpful because of the large range of symptoms of a nonspecific nature. Women have been told to snap out of it or have a baby or take a lover. Physicians have prescribed progesterone to alleviate symptoms, but double-blind studies by the NIH show that the hormone is no better than a placebo. Over-the-counter drugs are also of little value.

The one remedy that seems to help is exercise. When women do *moderate* exercise five times a week for at least thirty minutes a session, their symptoms are significantly reduced. If long, steady exercise causes a release of endorphins, it makes sense to keep the level "pumped up," so to speak, during the last two weeks of the cycle. Continuous production of endorphins makes withdrawal from the midcycle surge less likely to occur.

Exercise helps lessen symptoms. Dietary changes can also help reduce the intensity of the symptoms. For example, many women experience a craving for sweets and an increase in binging just before menstruation. But they also experience premenstrual weight gain, which leads them not to eat and to avoid sweets especially. Eventually the urge to binge may become uncontrollable, causing them to eat far more food, including sweets, than if they had eaten regular meals.

Research from the Massachusetts Institute of Technology suggests that there may be a link between serotonin in the brain and blood sugar. When blood sugar levels drop, serotonin is also low. This results in feelings of depression and the need to binge, both symptoms of PMS. (*Very* low levels of serotonin are seen in people suffering from the extreme effects of such symptoms: major depression and bulimia.) It's been shown that occasional small sugar snacks are effective in relieving the *milder* symptoms.

To avoid fluctuations in blood sugar (and possibly serotonin) levels, don't skip meals. Eat small frequent meals instead. Eat the same amount of food you normally would, but spread it out. Have three small meals and a midmorning and midafternoon snack.

It is better to limit simple sugars than to try to avoid them. It's okay to have some sugar, but don't have it on an empty stomach, for that could trigger a binge. Instead, have a dessert with your meal. It sounds strange, but it's better to eat dessert during the middle of a meal than at the end. Having something sweet at the end of a meal may lead you to want *more* sugar. If you eat the sweet midmeal, the craving is satisfied. Be sure to include fiber and protein with each meal to slow the digestion and absorption of the sugar.

Are these recommendations beginning to sound suspiciously familiar? You're right! Research now indicates that a low-fat, low-sugar, high-fiber diet is best for handling premenstrual syndrome. I wrote the *Fit or Fat Target Diet* just to help fat people lose weight. Now it's been shown that by following its principles you can combat heart disease, cancer, diabetes, and even PMS!

Additionally, limit your intake of caffeine and alcohol. Some women experience alcohol intolerance during the last two weeks of their cycle; they show signs of intoxication with only two drinks when it usually takes five or six to produce the same effects. Finally, sodium is not as big an issue as it once was, but if you're bothered by fluid retention and breast swelling or tenderness, then limit your sodium and avoid adding salt.

Fit Bones

IF YOU ARE FEMALE, white, fair-skinned, small-framed, and a smoker, you are at high risk for hip fracture, which is the second leading cause of accidental death for women aged forty-five to seventy-four. If you are over seventy-five, hip fracture is the *leading* cause of accidental death. One in five women who suffer from a broken hip will die of complications, such as pneumonia or blood clots in the lungs. One in two will never walk again. Some women get off lucky; they only go through months of pain and immobility, and never regain full function.

Older bones break primarily as a result of osteoporosis, a condition in which bone tissue is destroyed faster than it can be replaced. It occurs in women ten times as often as in men, with the greatest bone loss occurring during the five to seven years after menopause. By age sixty, most women have only three-quarters of the bone mass they had earlier. The most vulnerable areas are the wrist, the hip (what actually breaks in a hip fracture is not the pelvis but the top of the femur, the long leg bone that runs from the knee to the pelvis), and the spinal column. Osteoporotic women often have a series of small fractures of the vertebrae, which they sometimes interpret as bad backaches. These fractures result in compression of the spinal column and loss of height, sometimes as much as five inches. Or they may get "dowager's hump," a curvature of the spine at the shoulders.

The following risk factors increase a woman's chances of getting osteoporosis:

Alcoholism	Light frame
Sedentary lifestyle	Family history of osteoporosis
Cigarette smoking	Low calcium intake
Fair skin and hair	High protein intake
Childlessness	High phosphorus intake
Diabetes mellitus	

If you fall into two or more of these categories, you should be taking measures to avoid or at least reduce the severity of the disease. Osteoporosis cannot be cured, but physicians have had remarkable success in slowing down the degenerative process. Their approach is threefold: hormone therapy, diet, and exercise.

Estrogen is by far the most effective way to control osteoporosis. Estrogen can't restore bone that has already been lost, but it can prevent the accelerated loss that occurs during the first few years after menopause.

We have a dilemma here, don't we? The whole focus of this book has been on how to be low in fat, and taking female hormones drives fat levels up. Fat levels *do* increase with estrogen. Many women on estrogen therapy will gain 2–5 percent fat no matter how carefully they watch their diet and continue their exercise. Fortunately, laboratories have made some pretty dramatic changes in recent years with estrogen pills so that their product more closely imitates the estrogen produced by the body.

Younger women can take steps to further reduce their risk of osteoporosis. Getting adequate dietary calcium, of course, is one obvious step. In 1984 the NIH recommended an increase from a daily 800 mg. of calcium to 1000 mg. for premenopausal women and up to 1500 mg. per day for postmenopausal women. Research has since shown that taking extra calcium after menopause has less influence on bone loss than was thought. Even increasing calcium to 2000 mg. a day doesn't make a lot of difference. There *is* slightly less loss of the compact bone in hips and forearms, but no change in the rate of loss of spongy spinal bone. Again, the greatest positive effect on bone in postmenopausal women comes from the action of estrogen.

Rather than trying to ward off bone loss with supplements at menopause, women should make sure their diet always contains plenty of calcium-rich foods. (See the end of this chapter for a list of the calcium content of foods.) Your bones need a lifetime of care and attention. If you haven't supplied enough calcium to them for the last twenty or thirty years, you'll be entering menopause ill prepared for the "big storms" ahead. You can't "paint on" a coat of calcium at the last minute and expect it to do much good.

The other change a woman can make to slow down or prevent osteoporosis is to exercise more. Young, growing bones show measurable increases in mass in response to heavy exercise and dietary calcium. Parents of young girls should encourage their active participation in sports as well as supervise their diet to ensure that they are getting adequate calcium. By exercising and getting enough calcium, a young woman at maturity will achieve maximum bone growth and density.

After the skeleton has reached maturity, around twenty-five years of age, heavy exercise does little to augment bone mass. Unless you are an athlete who trains for hours a day, it would be impractical to try to increase bone mass. However, moderate exercise does protect against fractures. Exercise stimulates the activity of the osteoblasts, the cells that make bone, while slowing down the osteoclasts, the cells that break down bone. Thus, while not growing larger, bone may become denser. Additionally, exercise increases muscle mass, and a heavier layer of muscle better protects bones when falls occur. People who have regularly exercised throughout their lives have fewer bone fractures than those who haven't. They are more agile and use their muscles better to keep from falling.

What kind of exercise is best? I used to assume that you would have to do weight-bearing exercises to get calcium benefit, but studies have shown that *any* exercise that tugs and pulls on bones stimulates increased calcium deposition. In essence, when bone is constantly subjected to a "tug-of-war," demineralization is slowed and recalcification speeded up.

Because of the variety of exercises, I am inclined to favor aerobic dance classes for the prevention or delaying of osteoporosis. More women than men get osteoporosis, and more women are attracted to aerobic classes. They offer a nice balance of weight-bearing activity combined with floor exercises that pull and tug on the bones. For the woman who has beginning or advanced osteoporosis, a repetitive activity such as running may be detrimental. She should seek out classes that don't do too much of the same thing, are of low to moderate intensity, and include stretching and back exercises.

Calcium Content of Foods

100 mg.

Cottage cheese, ½ cup
Nonfat dry milk, 1 tbsp.
Cheese pizza, 1 section
Raw oysters, 8
Shrimp, canned, 3 oz.
Tofu, 3 oz.
Most nuts, 1 cup
Most dried beans and
   legumes, cooked, 1 cup
Corn muffin, 1
Dates, chopped, 1 cup
Raisins, seedless, 1 cup
Bok choy, ½ cup
Broccoli, 1 stalk
Spinach, ½ cup
Turnip greens, ½ cup
Mushrooms, 1 cup
Blackstrap molasses, 1 tbsp.

200 mg.

Most cheeses, 1 oz.
Ice cream or ice milk, 1 cup
Macaroni and cheese, 1 cup
Salmon, 3 oz.
Mustard greens, 1 cup
Collard greens, ½ cup
Kale, 1 cup
Creamed soups (mushroom, chicken,
   tomato), canned, prepared with
   equal amount of milk, 1 cup

300 mg.

Milk: nonfat, low-fat, whole,
   chocolate, or buttermilk, 1 cup
Ricotta cheese, ½ cup
Swiss cheese, 1 oz.
Yogurt, fruit-flavored, 1 cup
Pudding or custard, 1 cup

400 mg.

Yogurt, plain low-fat, or nonfat,
   1 cup
Milkshake, 10 oz.
Sardines, 3 oz.

What on Earth Is Brown Fat?

THERE ARE MILLIONS of fat cells in the body. Surgeons cut through vast numbers of them during practically every operation. When they are exposed to the human eye, most fat cells appear yellow in color.

There is an exception, however. There are very small clusters of fat cells that are brown in color. These clusters are so small that they can't be seen with the naked eye. In fact, a surgeon might cut through an area of brown fat without even knowing it. When they are observed under a microscope, they appear very similar to clusters of grapes, and we can see that the brown color is caused by a uniquely rich supply of both capillaries and nerve endings that pass through these fat clusters.

Clusters of brown fat are found in the chest, next to the spine, and around the blood vessels that lead to the heart. Brown fat cells are interesting because they work like little furnaces, burning fat and producing heat like crazy. They can consume a lot of calories, and, in some lucky people, turn excess calories into heat so that these excess calories are not stored as fat in the regular yellow fat cells. The yellow fat cell is rather passive, storing fat the way a squirrel stores nuts. There is very little metabolic burning of fat in yellow fat cells.

Brown fat, long ignored because there is so little of it, is creating big excitement in the research on obesity. It seems that brown fat cells can be activated to burn off vast quantities of calories in some individuals.

Athletic people occasionally eat 2000 to 3000 calories in excess of their body requirements without any increase in body fat. Researchers, using cameras, clocks, and notepads followed a group of athletes around for days to calculate their caloric requirements. For example, a 160-pound male might play tennis for two hours, four times a week. He might jog thirty minutes on each of the off days and square dance on Thursday nights. From this type of information the researchers might calculate that, on his average day, he requires 2500 calories.

Researchers might also keep track of the individual's food intake and determine that his normal intake is 2500 calories per day. In other words, this athlete seems to take in and burn off 2500 calories per day with no weight change. But once in a while, this individual eats as if it were Thanksgiving. On such "pig-out" occasions he may consume 6000 calories, 3500 of which are not needed and should result in an extra pound of fat. But they don't. In this athlete the extra calories stimulate or "turn on" increased heat production in the brown fat, so they are, in effect, wasted.

If you are fat, you may be bursting with joy. Don't get excited, because this doesn't seem to work if you are a fat nonexerciser. To explain this we need to look at the physiological chain of events:

1. Excess eating by the athlete stimulates the hypothalamus in the brain.
2. The hypothalamus sends nerve impulses to the brown fat, triggering the nerve endings to release noradrenaline.
3. Noradrenaline stimulates mitochondria in the brown fat to remove all of those excess calories from the pig-out. These calories are burned up, providing heat, but no fat storage.

This chain of events doesn't seem to apply to out-of-shape people. We don't know why. Maybe they have too little brown fat. We just don't know, because there is no practical way to test the amount of brown fat, its placement, or even its activity level in humans. Maybe out-of-shape people have enough brown fat but it doesn't function properly. Or maybe, because of continuous overeating (compared to their exercise level), their brains no longer respond to stimuli and therefore send no signals to the brown fat telling it to "light its burners." All we know is that when brown fat is properly stimulated, it increases in activity.

We also know that getting cold can turn on brown fat. The question is, if one gets cold often, will it stimulate brown fat to be increasingly responsive to cold? The functioning of most body mechanisms can be increased if used often, so it is tempting to assume that the brown fat mechanism can also be heightened with increased use.

A third peculiarity of brown fat is that it seems to be associated with exercise. Athletes have a more responsive brown fat mechanism, and as people become more athletic, the mechanism improves. It is not really clear which exercise stimulates brown fat the most. We may learn that long-distance running, or aerobics, or weight lifting is best. For the present, however, we can only observe that brown fat activity is higher in athletic people. At this point we can't even be sure that it is exercise itself that stimulates brown fat. It may be that exercise works only as an adjunct to cold and food.

The little clusters of brown fat cells are individually so small that you can't see them. But if the many clusters were grouped together and held in the hand, it would seem as if a new organ had been discovered in the body.

Researchers don't even know the real purpose of brown fat. We do know that it produces heat by consuming large quantities of calories. Perhaps this heat is just a by-product of the true purpose of brown fat. Some researchers feel that its location in the chest indicates that the main function is to heat the blood as it returns to the heart, but that is only a hypothesis at this point.

Now that you know brown fat can remove large quantities of calories from the blood, the next logical question is, "How can I make sure that my brown fat is working?" And, "How can it be stimulated so that I can eat anything I want without fear of storing the excess calories?"

A discussion of studies that have been done on animals might help us to better understand how eating, cold, and exercise can stimulate brown fat. Most of the research on brown fat to this point has utilized mice and rats. There is a highly inbred strain of mouse known as the "genetically obese mouse." This strain of mouse always becomes obese if fed all the food it wants. Although there appears to be a normal amount of brown fat in these animals, the usual stimuli of excess food and/or cold do not produce the fat-burning response because of a genetic malfunction in the brown fat cells themselves. This animal is very sensitive to cold; it will die if exposed to 40 degrees Fahrenheit (4 degrees Celsius) for only thirty minutes. This mouse's brown fat does not "turn on" in response to cold. However, the mouse does have a nervous system response. Its sympathetic nerves liberate noradrenaline in the brown fat tissue. Its brown fat mitochondria, however, don't respond to the noradrenaline. The mouse has brown fat. It seems to have all of the nerves to the brown fat. For some unknown reason the connection doesn't seem to work as it should.

Injecting noradrenaline early in life before obesity or cold sensitivity have developed has no effect on the genetically obese mouse. The brown fat cells still fail to turn on, proving that it is definitely a genetic defect.

There is also a genetically obese rat, which has a slightly different brown fat malfunction. This rat is not cold sensitive; it can turn on its brown fat when exposed to cold. The brown fat cells will not, however, turn on to increased food. In this animal noradrenaline injected into brown fat cells does stimulate increased heat production. It seems that their brown fat cells function quite well. But exposure to excess food doesn't trigger the sympathetic nervous system to produce noradrenaline. In this rat the defect seems to be in the central nervous system, which reacts to cold but not to excess food.

It seems possible that various combinations of the defects that have been found in the mouse and rat studies could be the culprit in those humans whose obesity is particularly stubborn.

The brown fat in children seems to function very well. When your house is chilly at 2 A.M., do your three-year-old children pull up more blankets the way you do? No, in fact they have probably kicked them onto the floor. It's natural for parents to want to add blankets to keep their children warm, but it may not be necessary. Their brown fat mechanism probably works better than yours, so in most cases they aren't cold, even if you are.

In essence, little kids may be turning up their heat production instead of putting on a blanket. The implication is that they are burning more calories. This is the probable explanation of the so-called "hollow leg." Young people can occasionally eat 1000 calories beyond the 2000 to 3000 they need and never gain an ounce. The extra calories go to the brown fat, where they are burned up.

As we get older, we are more likely to put on a coat rather than shiver in the cold. As a result, our brown fat cells may get lazy. They no longer try to burn fat (produce heat) because we don't ask them to. We avoid exercise and drafts because we chill easily. It's almost as if we are trying our best to decrease our brown fat cell activity.

Maybe adults could take advantage of cold weather to take a nice walk outdoors without the bundles of clothing they normally wear. If you get a bit cold you might possibly burn some excess calories and lose some weight. In fact, maybe we should expose ourselves to all of the conditions that are associated with good brown fat function: cold, occasional pig-outs, and exercise.

Since this research is in its infancy, it is probably premature for me to give advice. But I will tell you what *I* am going to do. I am going to try to stimulate my brown fat in every way I can. I will exercise a lot and expose myself to outdoor cold. Maybe it will be proven someday that brown fat activity decreases with age or that the sympathetic nervous system responds less well with age. If that is the case, I want to enter that phase of my life as well prepared with as much active brown fat as possible.

MOTIVATION

What Does Fitness Really Mean?

WHEN A FRIEND SAYS he has a cold and doesn't feel well, you may sympathize, but you know that he could be worse. If that friend develops pneumonia, your concern is greater. If you sprain an ankle, it may hurt like the dickens, but if you keep the weight off your foot for a few days, it will heal. If you break that ankle, you need more than just rest — you need a doctor to repair it. Many older people have ailments or body functions that don't work right. Maybe they are losing their hearing or their food doesn't seem to taste good anymore. If you ask them whether they feel sick, they may say no. But do they feel great? Another no.

My point is that there are stages or levels of being sick, and they aren't necessarily related to how much pain or discomfort you feel. A victim of an automobile accident may have an awful lot of pain, but you wouldn't say he was sick. In contrast, a person with heart disease may be very sick but not feel much pain. In other words, you can be sick and not know it — no pain, no symptoms. Sickness seems to be at the opposite end of the scale from health, with many degrees in between.

↑	5	Feel O.K.
Healthier	4	Malaise
	3	Trauma
Sicker	2	Degenerative disease
↓	1	Overt sickness

The scale on the previous page is one way to look at the different levels of sickness. The trouble with the scale is that it focuses on levels of feeling bad, omitting the levels of feeling good. After all, it's one thing to "feel O.K.," with nothing wrong that you can tell your doctor about, and it is another thing to feel great. The health/sickness scale should be expanded to include levels of *wellness*, as in this diagram.

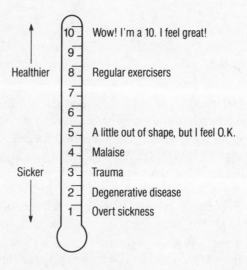

In the past physicians traditionally dealt with people at the bottom of the scale only. People who felt great didn't usually go to the doctor. The healthiest — or least sick — person a physician saw might have been a 6 or a 7.

However, as the nation got on its health kick, athletes went to doctors to become super-healthy. The concept was born that you could be more than "just O.K."; a person could enjoy a level of health that was formerly not even recognized. The indicators doctors used to appraise levels of health and sickness went off the top of their scales when they measured athletes. Athletes now get the highest health scores rather than those who used to be considered healthy. It is no longer true that health is the absence of feeling sick. It isn't enough to feel O.K. People want to feel great! It is characteristic of athletes that their bodies resist fatigue and the common complaints of the average person. In short, they are healthier than those who used to be considered healthy.

This idea that athletes are *very healthy people* seems obvious to us now, but it wasn't the normal way of thinking just a few years ago. Nutritionists have shifted the focus of their studies to athletes. Maybe, they said, if we study what these super-healthy people are eating, we will learn something new. And they did. They have learned that sugar, for example, is not quite as bad as we had thought. When fit people eat sugar, they *don't* get an insulin rush, and the sugar is turned into muscle glycogen for tomorrow's run. When out-of-shape people eat sugar, they convert it to fat and store it in their favorite fat cells. The point is, if you are really, really healthy your body handles sugar with no problems. People who "feel O.K." but are only 6's or 7's *are not super-healthy* and cannot handle sugar as well.

I don't want to get sidetracked into a discussion of sugar. My point here is that research is finding startling information about athletes. Fitness implies more than athletic ability — it implies a superior metabolism or body chemistry. The higher the level of fitness, the greater the body's control of all its parameters. Fitness, then, means being super-healthy.

What Your Doctor Should Know

FIFTEEN YEARS AGO, when I started lecturing, research had proven perhaps three medical benefits of exercise. Today medical opinion accepts more than *thirty* healthy changes brought about by exercise. Some changes are in tissues and organs directly affected by specific diseases, so some of the more forward-thinking doctors include exercise as an integral part of their treatment plans.

Exercise, particularly aerobic exercise, demands much of the body, stimulating physiological adaptations so that the body can handle the exercise better and better. We used to call the process simply "getting in shape." Now we realize that "getting in shape" implies a whole lot more. As people get in shape, there are improvements in their lungs, heart, muscles, and practically every other organ.

Picture your muscles as the motors of the body, much like the engine in your car. Without them nothing moves. You could not move your chest to pump your lungs, make your heart beat, or move a single finger. These motors need fuel and oxygen, just as a car does. Furthermore, like a car motor, they must expel an exhaust gas, carbon dioxide. To keep up with the demands of these motors during exercise, the lungs, heart, and circulatory system must work harder. Fortunately for us, these supply organs adapt to the demand put upon them.

As one becomes fit, muscles change so that they can use fuel and oxygen more efficiently, thus decreasing the work of the heart and lungs. You may feel that your lungs and heart are stronger after only a few weeks of exercise, but this feeling actually comes from muscle changes. Muscle improvements can be measured within days of starting an exercise program, while measurable improvements in heart function may take years. It's the skeletal muscles that control the body, not the other way around. If you make your motors work, they demand performance from all the supply organs. Almost every organ and tissue makes healthy changes if the muscles request it.

The medical advantages of aerobic exercise are so varied that it is hard to remember them all, so I have a gimmick. This gimmick might be a help to you when the time comes to relate this material to a fat friend. I draw a circle on a sheet of paper, or on a blackboard if I am lecturing. This circle represents the blood flow. Then I add little pictures to represent the organs that are affected by exercise. I put the brain at the top, since that's where it usually is, and the muscles at the bottom, because the best aerobic exercises always use the big muscles in the lower part of the body.

One effect of exercise on the brain is to change sleep patterns. In fit people a greater part of sleeping time is spent in the deeper and more restorative stages called Stage 4 sleep (virtual oblivion) and REM (rapid eye movement) sleep, when dreaming occurs. Fit people and wild animals seem to sleep so deeply that they feel restored with fewer hours of sleep. Perhaps you can remember awakening some mornings with the feeling you hadn't slept, even though you were in bed for seven or eight hours. You probably had a shallow, nonrestorative, unsatisfying sleep. In other words, not all hours of sleep are the same. Along the same line, one of the ways exercise helps alleviate depression is through deep sleep. Depressed people typically sleep fitfully. They awaken often during the night and usually have difficulty going back

AEROBIC EXERCISE AFFECTS EVERY TISSUE IN THE BODY

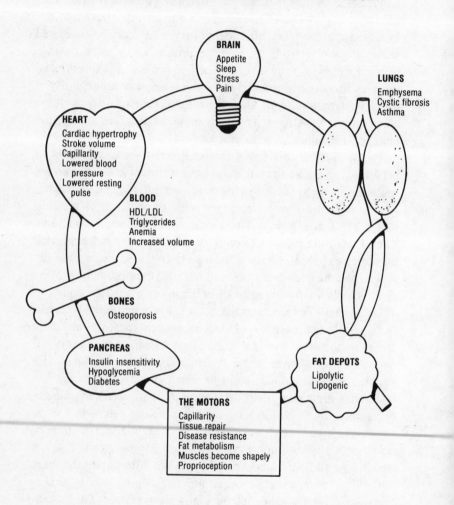

BRAIN
Appetite
Sleep
Stress
Pain

LUNGS
Emphysema
Cystic fibrosis
Asthma

HEART
Cardiac hypertrophy
Stroke volume
Capillarity
Lowered blood
  pressure
Lowered resting
  pulse

BLOOD
HDL/LDL
Triglycerides
Anemia
Increased volume

BONES
Osteoporosis

PANCREAS
Insulin insensitivity
Hypoglycemia
Diabetes

FAT DEPOTS
Lipolytic
Lipogenic

THE MOTORS
Capillarity
Tissue repair
Disease resistance
Fat metabolism
Muscles become shapely
Proprioception

to sleep. Long sessions of regular exercise help them go to sleep and stay asleep.

Hunger is also affected in several ways by exercise. When a fit person runs, fat cells release fatty acids, which slightly acidify the blood. Acid blood turns off hunger. On the other hand, when out-of-shape people exercise, their blood sugar often drops, which seems to increase hunger. Appetite is controlled by unconscious centers in the brain, which are often overruled by the conscious centers. As people get stronger, their physical strength seems to impart an emotional strength to the conscious centers. It is easier to say no to chocolate cake when you feel physically pumped.

Another effect of exercise on the brain is that it triggers the release of endorphins, which decrease pain. Everyone reacts differently to these painkillers so it's hard to pinpoint the mechanism, but endorphins *are* released during exercise and *may* be involved with relief from PMS, cramps, and stress.

If we move on to the lungs, we find that exercise has an effect on cystic fibrosis that is dramatic enough to energize the most skeptical physician. Among its many bad effects, cystic fibrosis causes scarring in the lungs. To my knowledge, no drug, no treatment plan, nothing slows the scarring process as effectively as exercise. Less dramatic, but important to a broader group of people, is the effect of exercise on the lung airways, the bronchioles. In fit people these tubes dilate more, so that air passes in and out of the lungs more quickly. In asthmatics the bronchioles constrict at the wrong time because the little muscles surrounding them are sort of spastic. I'm not saying that exercise cures asthma, only that exercise has a good effect on the little muscles that work improperly in asthmatics.

Next on my diagram are fat depots, those places on the body where fat cells predominate. The fat-cell changes caused by exercise are roughly opposite those caused by fasting. If you starve a fat cell, it retaliates by gearing up its fat-*storing* (lipogenic) mechanism. In contrast, the fat-*releasing* (lipolytic) mechanism picks up if you exercise regularly. Given these fat-cell changes, how can a physician not push exercise if he honestly wishes to help a fat patient? How can he tell the patient that her metabolism is slow but omit the fact that exercise is the only way to achieve a long-lasting increase in metabolism? How your fat cells behave makes a great difference in your tendency to get fat. Each living fat cell has a "mind" of its own. It's not important how many you have, it's what they are doing that counts. Do they release fat well or store it well? At 7 A.M. I run with my doctor so we can keep our fat cells in shape. Is your doctor having coffee and doughnuts at that hour?

Muscles respond to exercise particularly quickly. To *you* this means increased shapeliness in your legs, buttocks, and whole body. To *Covert Bailey* this means a higher rate of fat metabolism. To the *professional athlete,* muscle changes mean better proprioception. That is the athlete's inner sense of body control, which allows the figure skater to do unbelievable stunts and the boxer to know exactly how far he needs to reach to punch his opponent. To your *doctor,* muscle changes mean an increase in capillaries. As the number of capillaries increases, blood pressure drops. A woman who is not overweight is approximately 32 percent muscle. You can imagine that if 32 percent of your body has an easier blood flow, your heart has a lot less work to do. Changes in the number of capillaries and in blood flow also affect your body temperature and the rate of wound repair, clearly factors that are of interest to your doctor.

Exercise even affects the pancreas, although somewhat indirectly. The pancreas produces insulin when we eat sugar or, for that matter, almost any carbohydrate. In fit people, less insulin is needed to handle the blood glucose produced from carbohydrates. If you have diabetes in your family history, it will pay you to keep fit so that the demand on insulin production is not so great.

The pancreas also produces glucagon, which releases glucose from the liver when blood sugar is low. Because fit people use fat for fuel, their blood sugar is less likely to be low (hypogly-

> Exercise is good medicine.

cemia), and this in turn lessens the demand for glucagon from the pancreas. I have greatly simplified these complex relationships; I can assure you that competent endocrinologists know much more about them than I do. Nonetheless, they dare not leave exercise out of their deliberations.

Moving on around my diagram, we come to bones. I won't discuss them here because the chapter "Fit Bones" is devoted to that subject.

Blood, too, shows some pretty dramatic exercise-induced changes. One of the most amazing changes is in cholesterol. There are two kinds of cholesterol: high-density lipoprotein (HDL) and low-density lipoprotein (LDL). HDL is considered a "safer" form of cholesterol in that it doesn't tend to stick to arterial walls and may, in fact, actually reduce cholesterol deposits.

Ideally, at least 25 percent of your cholesterol should be of the HDL type. Premenopausal, sedentary women seem to average about 31 percent HDL. But this advantage is lost with menopause, which is one of the reasons why older women have the same incidence of coronary artery disease as men do. Exercise does not seem to reduce *total* blood cholesterol; instead it increases the good HDL in the blood and decreases the bad LDL. Women who have had endurance training average 39 percent HDL. If improvement in the HDL/LDL ratio were the only good thing about aerobic exercise, that in itself should be enough to get your doctor talking about it!

Aerobic exercise additionally helps prevent the formation of blood clots. In people whose blood vessels are already diseased and partially blocked with fatty cholesterol deposits, the possibility of thrombosis (blood clots in the deep veins of the legs) is great. If these clots break loose, they can travel to the lungs (pulmonary embolism), or the heart (myocardial infarction), or the brain (stroke). Sudden death is too often the final result.

A protein in blood, fibrin, is responsible for making the gelatin-like strands that give clots a solid structure. What stops fibrin from turning *all* of your blood into one big clot? The answer is that the cells lining blood vessels produce an enzyme called tissue plasminogen activator (tPA), which helps dissolve the fibrous strands. Physical activity stimulates production of tPA. Inactivity reduces output. If you're fat, you don't produce much tPA; if you're lean, you do.

Exercise helps prevent clot formation in another way. Fit people have more plasma, the liquid part of blood. Increased plasma means the blood isn't as thick and can move more smoothly through vessels. This more dilute blood is also less likely to form clots. If blood proteins, particularly fibrin, are diluted, the possibility of clots is decreased. In sedentary people the blood has a thicker composition, which encourages clot formation. People who have seldom exercised are sometimes reluctant to start because they figure it's too late to do any good. While it *may* be true that the fatty plaques formed in atherosclerosis are irreversible, it isn't too late to prevent or significantly delay the production of obstructive clots that cause the actual heart attack or stroke.

Exercise induces many changes in the heart, some of which have been known for a long time. For example, the heart enlarges, a condition called cardiac hypertrophy. Before athletes were studied so intensely, doctors often saw enlarged hearts in patients with passive heart failure, in which case the enlargement was a bad sign rather than a good one. More than one physician has confused an athlete's enlarged heart with a pathological enlarged heart. In long-distance athletes, an enlarged heart is the norm and is a great advantage in that it increases the volume of blood that can be pumped. Additionally, athletes have more capillaries in their heart muscles, which reduces the danger from heart attack.

Even this abbreviated list of health benefits resulting from exercise is impressive, and new benefits are being discovered all the time. Exercise is the miracle drug of the century. It is the elixir of life. Exercise has more positive medical effects on body organs than any drug or medical treatment plan ever devised. If your doctor doesn't exercise and doesn't urge you to exercise, he or she is neglecting the best medical advice available.

How to Be As Sleek and Low Fat As a Deer

SUPPOSE YOU WANT to lose fat. You've noticed that wild animals and athletes are low in fat. So you start exercising and you lose no fat. Why? Well, wild animals and athletes are low in fat, but low fat is only one of their many characteristics. As we pointed out in the last chapter, exercise, or physical play, has many effects on the body, only one of which is to make it lose fat.

To exercise efficiently, the body must have all its parts working well, not just its fat level. You start an exercise program so that you can look like a deer, but your body says, "I will have to fix the hemoglobin level first." Then it might proceed to clear out your lungs. I don't mean to imply that there is any conscious thought behind all this. The body just seems to know what it wants to fix first, and efforts to direct this process seem to be fruitless. An athlete doesn't usually think about what is happening any more than kids or wild animals do. The athlete simply does his sport, gets fit, and his body fat goes down.

Too many people concentrate on fat, not realizing that other great things are happening in their bodies. To speed up the loss of fat, they cut calories too far, depriving their bodies of the nutrients needed to take care of the other parameters. They may lose

> I will make you a promise.
> If you continue to exercise aerobically,
> there *will* be improvement in your fat metabolism.
> I don't know how long it will take.
> I don't know how strong the effect will be.
> But you *will* get fat less readily.

weight, but they see little or no improvement in their athletic performance, and the body never gets around to actually *fixing* the control mechanism for maintaining low fat. In other words, you can't force the process too much — it all takes time.

Everyone knows the saying, "A chain is only as strong as its weakest link." Body fitness is like that. All of the links, or parameters, must work together for the whole system to function perfectly. And you usually can't tell which one is functioning the worst. As you start to get fit, the body responds by fixing the parameter that it wants to fix first. You may not get the immediate weight loss you expect because your body is fixing a whole bunch of other parameters. So don't worry if you can't lose weight right away. You may be like an old beat-up jalopy; everything needs fixing. Let your internal mechanic decide what to fix first.

Fat people can't picture their fat as having anything to do with health. I don't blame them, really. They gain and lose fat without noticing any overt signs of illness. They don't feel much different, except for feeling angry about their looks. But body fat is definitely linked to health and, in turn, to athletic ability.

Fat is not an isolated substance stuck on the body that goes up and down with diet. It goes up and down with your general systemic health. Now it becomes clear why kids can keep their body fat down so easily. They exercise a lot without being aware of it. It is also clear why women who regularly go to exercise classes can hold their weight better than those who simply diet all the time. You CAN diet away some fat, but dieting CAN'T decrease

Read this out loud:
"I'm a fat-burning animal."
Doesn't that sound great?
Read it out loud again.

your tendency to get fat. No amount of dieting will make you into a wild animal. Women who exercise aren't keeping their weight down by burning extra calories. The exercise itself burns few calories. What is happening is that exercise changes body chemistry (metabolism) in such a way as to favor a light body.

We see this particularly well in those wild animals that run for survival. Foxes, coyotes, deer — all maintain their weight and fat level even when kept in captivity. Their high level of fitness keeps their metabolism in a weight-losing mode for a very long time after they stop exercising. You can see the same thing in athletes. Long after they give up exercise, they don't gain weight. We see people who do almost no exercise, eat everything in sight, and gain no weight. They seem to have naturally low-fat bodies, but, when questioned, they admit that they used to exercise a lot. They are getting a residual effect from exercise just as wild animals do.

The Latest Social Error

A REPORTER ONCE ASKED me if the current exercise craze might be just another passing American fad, destined to fade away with the pet rock and the hula hoop. I don't think so. Americans may do a lot of crazy things, but we sure know how to make things work. We have one admirable trait in this country — if we find something that improves our lifestyle, we do it. Exercise fits that definition to a tee. It improves life physically, emotionally, and socially.

As health improves with daily exercise, so does your mental state, making life more fun and making you more fun to be with! People who claim they aren't interested in exercise or don't need to exercise are making more than a medical mistake; they are making a social error. They don't realize that people in the know are embarrassed by their attitude. It's almost like saying you don't care if your car runs badly, or you don't care if your house is falling down. If you haven't been exercising and you don't relish starting, don't admit it! In fact, do just the opposite — lie a little. Tell your friends all the good things that happen to *you* when *you* exercise. The more good things you say about it, the more appealing exercise will become. You can acquire a taste for it just as you can for a food you used to dislike. There is nothing like positive thinking, and exercise is the most positive health measure

I'm in training!
For what?
Oh, just training.
I'm thinking about
the mountains I'm going to climb,
the rivers yet to be paddled,
the square dance that lasts half the night.

known today. And after three or four months of regular exercise, you won't feel right without it. Your little lie will have become the truth.

The good effects of exercise are overwhelming. Those disparaging comments, articles, even books, which seek to put exercise aside as a waste of time are an insult to thinking people. "I-hate-to-exercise" books are not really funny; they are pathetic. Don't bad-mouth exercise. In today's society, it makes you look foolish.

What about Weight Control Clinics?

IT SEEMS THAT ALL of us occasionally wish that someone else would take over our lives for a while and let us escape from the never-ending chore of personal care and responsibility. If *I* have to control my chocolate chip cookie eating, I feel guilty about every one I eat, but I eat them anyway and feel out of control. If someone else directs me, as in childhood, I can enjoy, free of guilt, every cookie I get. The one-week weight loss places, often dubbed "fat camps," are ample testimony to the desire to escape our own decisions. Notice also the recent popularity of personal exercise counselors. On the surface, it seems absolutely ludicrous to hire someone to watch you pedal a stationary bicycle or walk on a treadmill, but people are doing it in increasing numbers. Are we trying to be kids again, return to the time when we couldn't even jump in the swimming pool without screaming, "Mom, Mom, watch me!"?

The truth is, PEOPLE NEED HELP. The flight to fat camps, weight loss centers, and personal coaches is a way of saying, "I CAN'T DO THIS BY MYSELF." It's sad, but the more difficult it is to lose weight, the greater the desire to escape the responsibility of thinking about it. Part of being an adult is having to make our own decisions. But to manage every minute of every day with intelligence and rationality is taxing. We need moments when we are free of that burden. We need the relief of giving in to temptations and treats that may not be good for us. If you are a woman, with the typical difficulty of keeping your fat level down, don't let anyone make you feel guilty about it. Your plea for help is *not* just the "want" of a child; it is the "need" of an adult. It seems that everybody needs help with fat control, and some people need it a lot.

People who go to fat camps often gain back the weight they lose. Most of them admit that such programs don't help, but they want to go back again next year. It's fun to give away your responsibilities for a while. Even the so-called medically supervised programs overlook the real problem. No amount of doctor talk or "behavior modification" is going to decrease what I call *the forever pressure of adultness*.

Most weight loss programs meet only once a week and rely on pills or formulated foods or injections. People do lose weight, but most gain it back. For people who have already tried almost everything and keep gaining back what they lost, there is a need for everyday support. They need someone to "be there" throughout the week's temptations. Once-a-week sessions leave them all alone for six long days in between. No matter how professional the counselor or authoritative the doctor, once a week doesn't cut it. It leaves too much free time for bad decisions.

It seems as if most people who go to weight control centers end up fatter than ever. Here is a frightening thought. Is it possible that the best way to gain weight is to go to a weight control center? I hope that isn't true. The point is that a very different approach is needed.

I believe that the basic ingredient of a good weight control program is to offer relief from *the forever pressure of adultness*. People have to be shown new ways of acting like a kid that are gratifying without being detrimental. In my weight control center, which we call the Fit or Fat Center, we take over people's decisions for a while, then lead them to self-directed, childlike, but healthy behaviors. It's a very concentrated program, still experimental, but I think we have found the secret.

Those who join one of the classes in our Fit or Fat Center are required to attend a minimum of an hour per day four times a week for three months. We only take people who live close by so that we can see them easily and often. We get to know practically everything about them, their kids, and their home life, so that our "rules" are practical and personal.

When a group starts, most of the time is spent in a classroom learning physiology and how to use the Target Diet. As the days and weeks go by, less time is spent in the classroom and more time on exercise. The participants find a natural bonding as they learn about each other and realize that they aren't completely alone, that other women have the same problems and insecurities. Our intent is to take away responsibilities for a while, then gradually give them back in a healthier form.

I'm sorry that my program is restricted to people in the immediate vicinity of Portland. You can't fly in and stay with us for a couple of weeks — it would defeat the whole purpose. In lieu of that, you will have to examine potential programs in your area with a newly critical eye. Before you start one, ask questions like these: Will the program leave me alone to make mistakes all week long and then dump a guilt trip on me at the once-a-week meeting? Do the program people realize that I already know what I'm doing wrong and what triggers it, or will they insult me by lecturing about the obvious? Will they give me what I really need, a little parenting all the time instead of a "big lecture" once in a while? And most of all, do they care about me six months, a year, three years from now? Do they know that no one ever finishes a proper weight control program, that the right program means new habits and new friends for a lifetime?

Women Who Are Afraid to Lose Weight

THERE ARE WOMEN who are afraid of losing weight! Their conscious mind says, "I want to lose weight," but their unconscious mind says, "No." Some of them are simply overcome by people's expectations of them when they are thin. After all, thin people are expected to do more, be more active. If I stay fat, people won't expect me to do much — it's a lot easier to watch television than play tennis.

One of the women in our weight loss center weighed 250 pounds when she started, dropped down to 200, then lost no more for several months. We tried to help her break through the plateau. Then one day she admitted that she had been cheating on the diet because she was afraid to go lower. She said, "If I go below 200, I will die." She explained that she'd always had a fat image of herself. She said, "I have always been a fat person even when I've been skinny. If I get skinny, my fat self won't exist anymore — I'll be gone, dead. I don't know who this new skinny person is, and I don't know how she should act. It's too scary to have to start life all over."

When she told this story to her group in our classroom, over half of the women shared similar feelings. One woman who is five pounds *under* her ideal weight claims also to have a fat self-image. She said, "I am a fat person. When I look in the mirror, I expect to see a fat person and I *do* see a fat person. It's true that I don't have fat on my hips and thighs right now, but it belongs there. Its absence is temporary. When people look at me, I'm sure they see a fat person because that is the image I project."

Another of our women, who has a beautiful face, admits that when she is thin she loses her privacy. People stare — and not just men. Women who were her friends start watching their husbands and act cold to her. What a two-edged sword beauty is — to be looked at, envied, desired, wanted, but to *feel* that you are hated.

Another woman in our group is afraid to lose weight because her husband then wants kinky sex. Her husband might argue that his sex is not kinky, that, rather, she is a prude. We don't question which of them is correct, because it isn't our job to decide right and wrong. Our job is to listen, understand, and care. Our instructors are taught to listen for the feelings and not to worry about whether they are well founded. One woman's sexual fear is another woman's fantasy. Fear based on reality or on neurosis is still fear, and it can create a tape recording in a woman's mind that prevents her from losing weight. Such a woman insists that weight loss is her primary motivation, but the tape recording keeps urging her to eat enough to maintain her weight. In any other weight loss program she would be considered a black mark. We allow her to keep her safety shield of fat while getting fit underneath it. We tell our customers that we will help them with weight loss — and we do. BUT we *really* want them to get fit so that they can better be whatever they want to be.

My seventeen-year-old daughter, who is beautiful, I believe, in more than her daddy's eyes, says that the number-two subject, after boys, on her girlfriends' minds is fat — fat thighs, and oh! these flabby legs! Apparently those ugly tape recordings of the mind have started already, urging these young girls to be someone else rather than be the best they can be. If fat and weight and weight control start to crowd the sensible part of a woman's mind so early, what hope have we who design weight control programs? There is a simple answer. Teach them to focus on their muscles, their chemistry, their metabolism — all those words that make up fitness. As women get fit, they get comfortable with themselves and they get healthy. In truly healthy women the ugly tape recordings — and the fat — simply go away.

How to Keep Motivated

STOP LISTENING to the *fat is ugly, women are doomed* talk. If a friend continues to bad-mouth exercise or to talk about dieting and her thighs all the time, warn her that you can't handle negative vibes anymore. Maybe give her two more chances, then move on to a healthier friendship. Avoid negative people.

Join or start a discussion group made up of women only. Talk about the things you do or the habits you have that seem to defeat your best exercise and diet intentions. You will soon realize that you are not alone in your feelings; you are "O.K."

Ask the group such questions as:

1. What demands do I make of myself that are unrealistic?
2. What are the triggers that put me off my diet?
3. What happened yesterday that prevented me from doing my intended exercise?
4. What does my boyfriend or husband do that defeats my intentions?
5. What would my boyfriend or husband be willing to do to help my intentions?

Don't let the group discussion deteriorate into bad-mouthing. Keep the conversation on things you can do to make yourself better.

Create a new image for yourself by making a list like this:

1. I am an exercise person.
2. I enjoy my daily exercise.
3. I don't like fatty foods.
4. I have my body fat tested occasionally because the bathroom scale doesn't really tell me anything.
5. I give my friends only three chances to stop bad-mouthing.

Include some of your personal goals on the list, such as attaining a realistic body fat level. If you need to lower your body fat by 10 percent, set a goal of losing 3 percent in six months. Put a copy of the list on your mirror and another on your dashboard. Read the list out loud twice a day.

If you can, form a discussion group to help each other make your lists realistic and then help each other stick with it. If you can't get a group together, find a buddy — not someone who commiserates with all your woes or who wants to tell you her problems. Find someone who is willing to be your mentor or conscience, who will memorize *your* list and bug you in a positive way to stay on track. If you think that no one wants to be in a group or be your mentor, you're probably not asking enough people. Even the woman next door, whom you may not know very well, shares your frustrations with body fat and will be pleased with your request. Remember, the tallest walls are the ones we build around ourselves.

Most important, don't overlook the man in your life. He is your closest ally, your best buddy. Yes, you are different from him. But in many ways you are very similar. What attracts you most to a man? His looks? His monetary value? His fame? Initially, these things may have piqued your interest, but in the long run you grow to love his inner qualities, his caring, his thoughtfulness, his devotion to you. Men, too, are attracted to beauty at first. It is a healthy, natural reaction to praise a beautiful sight, be it a woman or a sunset. But more than beauty, men applaud effort. They admire the woman who gets up a half-hour early to exercise, who joins in the basketball or volleyball game regardless of skill, who gets a kick out of making low-fat meals that taste like high-fat gourmet dishes. They like achievers.

Yes, women are different from men, emotionally, physically, and mentally. It's time for both sexes to enjoy the differences, be amused by them, and help each other when these differences cause problems. Men have emotions, too, and they sometimes say and do the wrong things. But they're willing to help you in any way they can, if you just let them.

It's time to let the new woman out, the woman who sets her own standards of performance and beauty. She is going to concentrate on her inner self, luxuriate when her muscles are sore, look forward to the feeling of strength, timing, and body sense. In her heart the new woman lives with the wild animals. It's all in the muscles — that's the secret of real beauty. Work those hidden beauties until they shine and ripple the fat away. It's muscles that make the tiger sleek and let the eagle soar.

The New Fit or Fat
revised and expanded version of the revolutionary best seller

The Fit-or-Fat Woman (with Lea Bishop)
on women's special weight and fitness problems

The Fit-or-Fat Target Diet
on designing your best diet

Fit-or-Fat Target Recipes (with Lea Bishop)
for easy, healthful meals

The Fit-or-Fat headquarters, now located near Portland, Oregon, continue to develop support material for professionals who want to be effective teachers of healthy lifestyles. Materials include books, audiotapes, videotapes, and seminars.

To schedule a lecture by Covert Bailey or to obtain a free copy of the newsletter which describes the Fit-or-Fat materials, write to:

Covert Bailey
P.O. Box 230877
Tigard, OR 97281

To order the Fit-or-Fat books, see your bookstore or phone 1-800-225-3362.

For multiple copies, phone the Houghton Mifflin Special Sales Department, 617-725-5969.